CLEFT PALATE

MIDDLE EAR DISEASE and

HEARING LOSS

CLEFT PALATE
MIDDLE EAR DISEASE and HEARING LOSS

Edited by

MALCOLM D. GRAHAM, M.D.
Associate Clinical Professor
Department of Otolaryngology
University of Southern California School of Medicine
Director
Otologic Electron Microscopy Laboratory
Ear Research Institute
Otologic Medical Group, Inc.
Los Angeles, California

with a Foreword by

Brian F. McCabe, M.D.
Department of Otolaryngology and Maxillofacial Surgery
University of Iowa Hospitals and Clinics
The University of Iowa
Iowa City, Iowa

and an Introduction by

D. C. Spriestersbach
Vice-President for Educational Development and Research
Dean of The Graduate College
Professor of Speech Pathology
Department of Speech Pathology and Audiology
Department of Otolaryngology and Maxillofacial Surgery
The University of Iowa
Iowa City, Iowa

THOMAS BOOKS SYMBOL OF LEADERSHIP

CHARLES C THOMAS · PUBLISHER
Springfield · Illinois · U.S.A.

CHARLES C THOMAS • PUBLISHER
BANNERSTONE HOUSE
301-327 East Lawrence Avenue, Springfield, Illinois, U.S.A.

ISBN 0-398-03667-5
Library of Congress Catalog Card Number: 77-3954

With THOMAS BOOKS *careful attention is given to all details of manufacturing and design. It is the Publisher's desire to present books that are satisfactory as to their physical qualities and artistic possibilities and appropriate for their particular use.* THOMAS BOOKS *will be true to those laws of quality that assure a good name and good will.*

Printed in the United States of America
N-1

Library of Congress Cataloging in Publication Data
Main entry under title:

Cleft palate: Middle ear disease and hearing loss.

Bibliography: p.
Includes index.
1. Middle ear—Diseases. 2. Cleft palate—Complications and sequelae. 3. Hearing disorders in children. I. Graham, Malcomb D., 1932-
[DNLM: 1. Cleft palate—Complications. 2. Ear, middle. 3. Ear diseases—Etiology. 4. Hearing disorders—Etiology. WV440 C626]
RF220.C57 618.9'209'784 77-3954
ISBN 0-398-03667-5

To
Dean M. Lierle, M.D., who provided the environment and stimulation for so many young men and women in many fields of interest to become involved in the care of the child born with a cleft palate.

Contributors

LESLIE BERNSTEIN, M.D., D.D.S.
Professor and Chairman
Department of Otorhinolaryngology
University of California,
Davis, California

CHARLES D. BLUESTONE, M.D.
Professor
Department of Otolaryngology
University of Pittsburgh School of Medicine
Director
Department of Otolaryngology
Children's Hospital of Pittsburgh
Pittsburgh, Pennsylvania

RICHARD A. BUCKINGHAM, M.D.
Clinical Professor of Otolaryngology
Abraham Lincoln School of Medicine
University of Illinois
Attending Otologist
Resurrection Hospital
Chicago, Illinois
Hines Veterans Administration Hospital
Hines, Illinois

MALCOLM D. GRAHAM, M.D.
Associate Clinical Professor
Department of Otolaryngology
University of Southern California School of Medicine
Director
Otologic Electron Microscopy Laboratory
Ear Research Institute
Otologic Medical Group, Inc.
Los Angeles, California

JACQUELINE KEASTER
Former Director
Hearing and Speech Clinics
Children's Hospital
Los Angeles, California

DANIEL LING, Ph.D.
Professor of Aural Rehabilitation
School of Human Communication Disorders
McGill University
Montreal, Canada

FRED H. LINTHICUM, M.D.
Director
Eccles Temporal Bone Laboratory and Larrabee Microscopy Center
Director of Education
Ear Research Institute
Associate Clinical Professor of Otolaryngology
University of Southern California School of Medicine
Otologic Medical Group, Inc.
Los Angeles, California

RALPH A. NELSON, M.D.
Assistant Professor
Department of Otolaryngology
Eastern Virginia Medical School
Norfolk, Virginia
Chief
Department of Otolaryngology
Naval Regional Medical Center
Portsmouth, Virginia

LARRY SEVEREID, M.D.
Clinical Instructor
Department of Otolaryngology
University of Wisconsin
Madison, Wisconsin
Gundersen Clinic Ltd.
La Crosse, Wisconsin

D. C. SPRIESTERSBACH
Vice-President for Educational Development and Research
Dean of The Graduate College
Professor of Speech Pathology
Department of Speech Pathology and Audiology
Department of Otolaryngology and Maxillofacial Surgery
The University of Iowa
Iowa City, Iowa

Foreword

A VOLUME SUCH AS THIS has long been needed in medicine. The identification and long-term treatment of middle ear disease and hearing loss in cleft patients is absolutely essential to their proper management. This fact is too frequently neglected by some cleft management teams, or otology is given a very secondary role in the activities of the team. If not excusable, this untoward event is in many ways understandable. The child's appearance cries for correction and may get the preponderance of attention. The child's speech, when rhinolalia aperta is present, is a constant reminder to all that this problem must be attended to vigorously. At the same time, middle ear disease and hearing loss may be subtle. The ears may not drain, a tympanic perforation may not be present or recognized, retraction may not be obvious, the evidence of middle ear fluid is questionable, and the child does not complain of hearing loss. He does not complain because he has grown accustomed to the stuffy feeling in his ears and issued to the 25 or 30 dB speech reception threshold that he has had now for many months or years. The net result is a child who appears and speaks reasonably or very well, is a poor communicator, fails to live up to his intelligence quotient in school, and develops suboptimally in both social and intellectual areas. This is because a child with a 25 or 30 dB hearing loss in each ear misses nearly one half of the information presented to his ears. Such a child cannot possibly develop maximally. The mounting evidence that chronic secretory otitis media is in most children a self-resolving disease may lead a team to disregard this disease to the detriment of the child. It is also true that some of these ears go on to develop cholesteatomatous disease and permanent partial deafness. Thus, a cleft child deserves and must have continuing audiologic evaluation and otologic care.

That is why this book is so important.

BRIAN MCCABE, M.D.

Preface

DURING THE PAST TWO DECADES, an increasing concern for the rehabilitation of the individual born with a cleft lip and/or palate has developed. The techniques of surgical repair have been well established, and the management of the speech handicap has received much attention. However, the hearing disability so frequently found in the child with the cleft palate has only recently received attention.

In preparing this book, the contributors have attempted to present their experience in a succinct fashion in the hope that the material contained in this volume will have wide appeal to those involved with the care of the cleft palate individual: otolaryngologists, plastic surgeons, pediatricians, speech pathologists, audiologists, dental specialists, educators, social workers, and psychologists. It is hoped that this book will be recommended reading in the undergraduate and graduate programs in these various disciplines.

We hope we have been successful in this task.

MALCOLM D. GRAHAM, M.D.

Introduction

THE DEPARTMENT OF OTOLARYNGOLOGY and Maxillofacial Surgery of the University of Iowa College of Medicine has played a pioneering role in documenting the prevalence of ear disease among persons with cleft palate and in establishing effective regimens for treating the disease. In part, this role was the consequence of the composition of the Department which included not only otolaryngologists but also plastic surgeons, speech pathologists, audiologists, dentists, social workers, nurses, and psychologists. In great measure, of course, the role was the consequence of the leadership and vision of the long-time head of the Department, Doctor Dean M. Lierle, who brought together the several specialists required for the total habilitation of individuals with cleft lip and palate and established a working milieu enabling each to function effectively with the others. In parts, too, the role was the consequence of the system of medical care in the State of Iowa granting families of children with clefts long-term care at the University of Iowa Hospitals without regard to their ability to pay for the care. Such a system made it possible for the patient to be seen from birth or shortly thereafter until all habilitative procedures had been completed.

Given the primary mission of the Department, it is not surprising that the condition of the ears of the patients with clefts were not overlooked during evaluation and treatment. Furthermore, it is not surprising that relatively large series of records of the otologic and audiologic evaluations of these patients at various age-levels and of the same patients over time were accumulated. These records produced a rich resource for study and reflection. As a consequence, those who received some or all of their training in the Department, especially the otolaryngology and maxillofacial residents, were sensitized to the potential hearing problems of the cleft population. In fact, it is presumable the person responsible for the preparation of this book, Dr. Malcolm Graham, found the stimulus for it during the time of his residency at Iowa. As a matter of fact, he used a portion of the ear histories of the Iowa patient series as the source of the data for his Master of Science thesis.

During the 1950s and early 1960s, I, too, was a member of the Iowa cleft palate group. In the course of that experience, I became convinced of the validity of the team approach in mounting an effective program of cleft palate habilitation. Not uncommonly, the concerns of the otologists over the pathological conditions of the patients' ears provided significant input in the development of our habilitation plans.

My purpose in citing the Iowa program and my experience with it is not meant to be self-serving. Other cleft palate teams developed as early as Iowa's and others were equally aware of the importance of ear disease among cleft palate populations. I have cited the Iowa history to establish my credentials for commending the authors of this book for undertaking the task of presenting the comprehensive story of this facet of the cleft palate problem. It deserves the attention of all specialists working with cleft patients, and it should do much to ensure that the ears of the patient with a cleft will receive as careful attention as the cleft itself.

D. C. SPRIESTERSBACH

Acknowledgments

THE EDITOR ACKNOWLEDGES with great appreciation the help of the contributors to this volume. Their contributions represent the experience of many years of working with the individual with a cleft palate, and I am most grateful for their willingness to share this experience.

To Mrs. Karon W. Hoffman and Ms. Annette Florance, my secretaries, I owe a very heavy debt of gratitude for their help in manuscript preparation. Mr. Lawrence E. Irwin helped with many technical details, and I am very appreciative.

My wife, Julia, and children, Scott, Cameron, Melissa, and David, understood the time this book required for preparation, and for their encouragement, I am most grateful.

M.D.G.

Contents

CLEFT PALATE
MIDDLE EAR DISEASE and HEARING LOSS

—1—

ANATOMY AND PHYSIOLOGY OF CLEFT PALATE

LESLIE BERNSTEIN, M.D., D.D.S.

CLEFT LIP AND PALATE is one of the most frequent congenital malformations. In addition to visible disfigurement and problems with chewing and deglutition, patients with this malformation find their disability compounded by the inability to communicate verbally with others in a socially acceptable manner.

THE ANATOMY OF THE NORMAL PALATE

The palate is made up of the primary palate, or *premaxilla,* and the secondary palate, which is the major portion of the palate posterior to the premaxilla, consisting of most of the hard palate and all of the soft palate (Fig. 1-1).

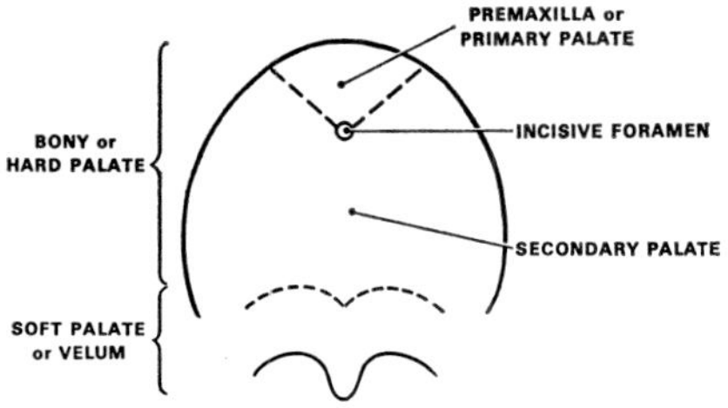

Figure 1-1. Topographic areas of the palate. From L. Bernstein, Congenital Defects of the Oral Cavity. In M.M. Paparella and D.A. Shumrick (Eds.): Otolaryngology, Vol. III, *Head and Neck,* 1973. Courtesy of W.B. Saunders Company, Philadelphia, Pennsylvania.

The Hard Palate

The hard palate consists of the premaxilla, the palatine processes of the maxilla, and the horizontal plates of the palatine bones. A midline dehiscence immediately behind the incisor teeth, the incisive foramen, is the point of division between the primary and secondary palates. The incisive foramen leads obliquely in a posterosuperior direction into the nasal cavity and is divided into a left and right portion by the overlying nasal septum. An irregular suture line, extending from the incisive foramen to the alveolar process between the lateral incisor and canine teeth, outlines the premaxillary segment. The greater palatine foramen lies posteriorly, on the medial aspect of the alveolar process, between the palatine bone and the maxilla; the lesser palatine foramina are located a little further back.

Anteriorly and along its median third, the palate is covered by a mucoperiosteum which is strongly adherent to the underlying bone and may be separated from it only with some difficulty. Posterolaterally, the intervening space between the mucous membrane and the periosteum is widened to contain mucous glands.

The hard palate receives its blood supply from the greater palatine artery, which emerges from the greater palatine foramen and curves forward, assuming a lateral relationship to the accompying greater palatine nerve. This artery enters the incisive foramen and supplies the anterior portion of the floor of the nose and lower part of the anterior nasal septum. The venous drainage is posteriorly into the pterygoid plexus. Other veins ramify in the superior tonsillar region and join the pharyngeal plexus. The lymph drainage is to the retropharyngeal and deep cervical lymph nodes.

The nerve supply of the hard palate is derived from the greater palatine nerve, a branch of the maxillary nerve, and extends forward as far as the maxillary-premaxillary suture line. The area of the primary palate is supplied by the sphenopalatine nerves which enter the oral cavity through the incisive foramen.

Where the two horizontal processes of the palatine bones fuse in the midline along the posterior edge, they form a well-defined spine pointing backward, the posterior nasal spine.

The Soft Palate

Much of the bulk of the soft palate, or *velum,* is made up of mucous and serous glands present in its oral mucous membrane. On its oral aspect, the velum is covered with stratified squamous epithelium, which is continuous over its posterior border with the nasal surface. Stratified squamous epithelium is present on its nasal surface in the region where it comes into contact with the posterior pharyngeal wall. The oral epithelium contains only a few taste buds. The anterior portion of the nasal surface is covered by a ciliated pseudostratified columnar epithelium with many goblet cells. The uvula and the adjacent portion of the soft palate are occupied by large masses of mucous and serous glands with ducts opening onto the oral surface of the soft palate. Scattered lymphoid follicles may be found in the oral mucous membrane.

The blood supply of the soft palate is furnished by the lesser palatine branches of the maxillary artery and by the ascending palatine branch of the facial artery, together with palatine branches of the ascending pharyngeal artery. Venous drainage occurs laterally through the walls of the pharynx into the pharyngeal and pterygoid plexuses. Lymphatic drainage is into the retropharyngeal and anterosuperior deep cervical lymph nodes.

The soft palate receives its nerve supply from the maxillary division of the trigeminal nerve, reinforced laterally on the oral surface by the glossopharyngeal nerve. The maxillary nerve fibers arrive as the lesser palatine nerves through the sphenopalatine ganglion. Taste fibers pass through the greater superficial petrosal nerve to the nervus intermedius.

Functionally, the soft palate is a fibromuscular structure consisting of an aponeurosis acted upon by several muscles to produce alterations in its shape and position (Fig. 1-2). This aponeurosis consists of the flattened tendon of the tensor palati muscles which join in the midline to form a common sling.

The *tensor palati muscle* arises from the base of the skull and the lateral aspect of the cartilaginous part of the auditory (eustachian) tube. The origin extends from the scaphoid fossa at the upper end of the medial pterygoid plate along the greater wing of the sphenoid bone to the sphenoidal spine. From this origin, the

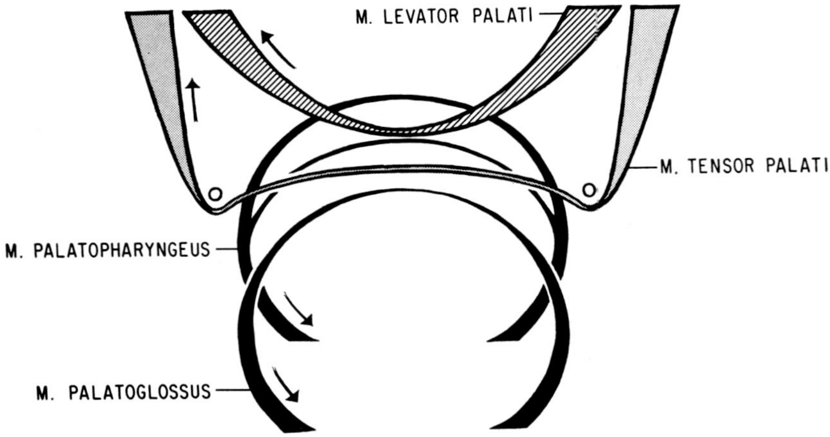

Figure 1-2. Diagrammatic representation of the sling action of the various muscles attached to the soft palate.

flat muscle extends medially and inferiorly, converging on the base of the hamular process of the sphenoid bone to become a flat tendon. This tendon passes above the fibrous arch of origin of the buccinator muscle and bends at right angles around the base of the hamulus to enter the pharynx. The tendon now widens into a broad triangular aponeurosis joining with its fellow on the opposite side. The aponeurosis is attached to the crest of the palatine bone. The posterolateral border blends with the side wall of the pharynx anteriorly and hangs free posteriorly to form the posterior border of the soft palate.

The uvula hangs as an appendage from the central portion of the soft palate. Although it contains the uvula muscle, its function is quite insignificant.

When the palatine aponeurosis becomes tense, it produces a flattening of the normal concave shape of the soft palate and a simultaneous downward depression. The main action of the tensor palati is to tense the aponeurosis so that other muscles may elevate and depress it without altering its shape. Another important function of the tensor palati muscle is the alteration of the normally vertically oriented long axis of the auditory tube opening into a horizontal orientation. This produces the snap opening of the tube. The tensor palati muscle is supplied by the motor division of the trigeminal nerve via the nerve to the medial pterygoid muscle and the otic ganglion.

The *levator palati muscle* arises from the quadrate area at the apex of the petrous temporal bone anterior to the carotid foramen. The muscle converges to form a rounded belly and is inserted into the nasal aspect of the palatine aponeurosis between the two heads of the palatopharyngeus muscle. Additional fibers of origin extend from the medial aspect of the auditory tube cartilage. The two muscles are directed anteriorly and medially, together forming a **V**-shaped sling which pulls the palate superiorly and posteriorly. The soft palate comes into contact with the posterior pharyngeal wall on a level with the anterior arch of the atlas vertebra. Contraction of the levator palati muscle opens the auditory tube in a manner similar to that following contraction of the tensor palati muscle. The levator palati muscle receives its nerve supply from the pharyngeal plexus, the nerve fibers arising in the cell bodies of the nucleus ambiguus and passing to the pharyngeal plexus by way of the accessory nerve and the pharyngeal branch of the vagus nerve.

The *palatopharyngeus muscle* has two heads of origin which embrace the insertion of the levator palati muscle on the nasal surface of the palatine aponeurosis. The anterior head arises from the posterior border of the hard palate. The palatine aponeurosis lies on its oral surface and passes forward to attach to the crest of the palatine bone. The posterior head arises from the superior aspect of the palatine aponeurosis. The two heads arch laterally and inferiorly over the lateral border of the aponeurosis to join and form a muscle belly constituting the posterior pillar of the fauces. The lower portion of the muscle is inserted into the posterior border of the ala and cornua of the thyroid cartilage. Additional fibers are inserted anteriorly into the superior border of the ala of the thyroid cartilage, while some blend posteriorly with fibers of the inferior constrictor muscle. The palatopharyngeus muscle is an elevator of the larynx and pharynx, arching the relaxed palate and depressing the tensed palate.

The nerve supply is similar to that of the levator palati

muscle, from the pharyngeal plexus by way of the pharyngeal branch of the vagus, which consists of accessory nerve fibers with their cell bodies in the nucleus ambiguus.

The *palatoglossus muscle* arises from the under surface of the palatine aponeurosis and passes downward to blend with the musculature in the side of the tongue. The body of the palatoglossus forms the anterior pillar of the fauces and has a sphincteric action at the oropharyngeal isthmus. It contracts to raise the tongue and narrows the transverse diameter of the oropharyngeal isthmus. It is innervated by the pharyngeal plexus in a similar fashion to the palatopharyngeus and levator palati muscles.

The *ridge of Passavant,* first described in 1869, is difficult to define anatomically in normal subjects; however, it may be readily visible in a patient with an unrepaired cleft palate. On swallowing, in cleft palate individuals, the posterior third of the soft palate moves toward the pharyngeal wall at the level of Passavant's ridge. It would appear that, both functionally and anatomically, the elevation of Passavant's ridge is a minor feature of the complex movements of swallowing. Disagreement exists whether to regard the musculature of Passavant's ridge as a portion of the superior constrictor muscle or as a portion of the palatopharyngeus muscle. Last[3] and others regard this latter view as being correct. Cinefluroscopic studies by Calnan,[2] demonstrating closure of the oronasal space by contact of the soft palate during speech with the posterior pharyngeal wall at a level 1 to 2 cm above Passavant's ridge, have disproved Passavant's original theory and verified Veau's skepticism of the function of Passavant's ridge.

SOFT PALATE ACTION IN SPEECH

Given an acceptable lip repair, speech is the most important function to consider in cleft palate management—a situation underscoring the need for cleft palate surgeons to receive some training in speech pathology. The major action of the soft palate during speech is concerned with the modulation of the velopharyngeal sphincter. Although the action is voluntary in the strict sense of the word, a major aspect of the action is unconscious and well coordinated with the pharyngeal and glossal musculature in the production of normal speech. The muscles responsible for closure of the velopharyngeal aperture are the levator palati muscles, aided by the stiffening effect produced by the tensor palati muscles. Velopharyngeal closure is also aided by the superior constrictor and perhaps also by the ridge of Passavant.

Velopharyngeal competence refers to the normal function of these muscles in the production of normal speech. On the other hand, velopharyngeal incompetence refers to the total or partial inability of these structures to shut off the nose from the oropharynx during speech production. The characteristic of the muscles concerned with controlling the velopharyngeal sphincter is that they are highly efficient, contract rapidly, and have a very quick recovery.

A competent speech mechanism is required for the production of normal speech. Although "normal speech" may be differently defined by individuals with varying attitudes to the subject, the expression does imply that competent velopharyngeal closure exists. With the exception of the consonant sounds "m," "n," and "ng," all other consonant sounds in the English language require the build-up of intraoral air pressure. The sudden release of this pressure produces an explosive sound, or a *plosive* consonant, such as "p," "t," and "d." The production of sound by friction produces *fricative* consonants, such as "f," "th," "v," and "z." The more silent fricatives are specified as *sibilants,* such as "s" and "sh."

When sounds are produced by individuals with velopharyngeal incompetence, they take on a nasal quality, more properly called *hypernasality.* This is in contrast to the hyponasality heard in obstructed conditions of the nasal airways, such as with a hypertrophied adenoid or a head cold.

When enunciated by patients with velopharyngeal incompetence, consonants are frequently distorted by inadequate pressure and/or by the sound of air leaking into the nose, referred to as *nasal escape.* Certain cleft palate individuals may learn to omit such sounds or to substitute for them with other sounds, such as those produced by building up pressure below the glottis and producing a plosive called a *glottal stop.* The word "daddy" then becomes "ah-ee" with the consonants omitted or close to "gha-ghee" with the glottal stop.

THE DEVELOPMENT OF CLEFTS

Palatal clefts are the result of failure of fusion of the mesodermal component of the particular segments. It is generally accepted that fusion of these segments takes place between the seventh and twelfth weeks of intrauterine life.

Congenital palatal clefts follow the lines of fusion of the various segmental components of the palate. Some knowledge of the embryology of the palate is, therefore, mandatory to the appreciation of palatal clefts and their related anomalies.

Phylogenetically and embryologically, the palate may be divided into two distinct regions. The triangular structure anterior to the incisive foramen and originating from the median nasal processes is the premaxilla, or the *primary palate.* Posterior to the premaxilla is the *secondary palate* which consists of the palatal processes of the maxillae, the horizontal laminae of the palatine bones and the velum, or *soft palate.* Overriding the outer perimeter of both the primary and secondary palates is the alveolar process, the ridge of the dental arch.

Stark studied six human embryos with cleft lip and cleft palate.[4] He found that the absence of mesoderm in the lip and premaxilla coexisted with the presence of a cleft in each instance. On the other hand, it is noteworthy that, in the region of the hard and soft palate, mesoderm was present upon each side of the cleft in approximately equal amounts, but this may be explained on the basis that these were midline clefts. In each of the six embryos studied, some mesoderm was always present in the lip-premaxillary region. However, when the mesoderm was absent unilaterally, a single cleft resulted; when it was absent bilaterally, a double cleft ensued. It is suggested from these studies that a lack or even a diminution in mesoderm will lead to the formation of a cleft in an area normally poor in mesoderm. These facts are not at variance with the theory of mesodermal penetration of a preexisting epithelial wall.

Moreover, a relative, as well as a total, lack of mesoderm may exist in a given area, which must account for the widely variable severity of these deformities. The theory of mesodermal penetration gains further credence by the presence in the occasional "partial" cleft lip case of a synechial band of tissue at the base of the nostril (Simonart's band), which is all that prevents the notch from becoming completely cleft. Such a band suggests that it is the sole remaining vestige of a fraying epithelial wall rather than the coapted edges of adjacent facial processes. Also suggestive of a distraction force is the presence of split supernumerary teeth on each side of the cleft, which occurs in most patients.

It is felt, therefore, that initially an epithelial anlage exists in the region that is to become the lip and that in this epithelial wall there are normally three masses of mesoderm: one placed centrally and the other two laterally. If any of these masses are absent or deficient, the wall will become attenuated, and a cleft lip will develop. The severity of the cleft bears a direct relationship to the amount of mesodermal deficiency.

The embryology of the associated premaxilla that develops with the lip also needs to be understood. Coincidental with the development of the upper lip is the development of its allied structures, namely, the nasal septum, prolabium, and premaxilla. These structures develop from the fourth to the seventh week, and the combined entity has been variously termed the primary palate, intermaxillary segment, intermaxilla, and prepalatal segment. As the nasal pits deepen, the oronasal membrane ruptures, forming the primitive posterior nasal choanae. The primitive nasal airways thus delineate the primary palate. As the palatal shelves rise and fuse, they do so beginning at these choanae, fusing progressively in a posterior direction. The incisive foramen remains as the vestige of the former posterior choanae, which is also the division between anomalies of the primary and secondary palates.

Behind the lip-premaxillary segment, the hard and soft palates develop together, but at a different time and in a different way from the primary palate. The hard and soft palates develop from the seventh to the twelfth weeks and together are termed the secondary palate. This forms from the palatine shelves or processes consisting of mesoderm surfaced with ectoderm. These processes are located posterior to the primitive choanae and hang obliquely downward alongside the tongue. Due to some inexplicable increase in tension, the shelves begin arching over the tongue at the eighth to ninth week. This elevation of the shelves occurs as a wave from front to back. When the elevation is completed, the palatal shelves begin to fuse together from the anterior to the posterior direction. The fusion is completed by the twelfth week. While this has been taking place, the nasal septum has been growing downward to meet the fusing palatal shelves.

Because the secondary palate develops according to the classic doctrine of fusion of processes, any impedance to development from the seventh to the twelfth week of gestation may interrupt the elevation and fusion of the palatine processes, producing a persistence of the original cleft in the roof of the mouth.

It has been shown that, in rodents, the right palatal shelf reaches the horizontal position before the left one, leaving the left side vulnerable to interruption or interference in its normal development for a longer period of time than the one on the right.[5] This may explain the more frequent occurrence of unilateral clefts on the left than on the right side in humans.

Although experimental clefts have been produced in animals by a variety of insults, notably the steroids, these clefts are not genetically reproducible. In humans, the only known cause of clefting is heredity. This certainly applies to the most common type of cleft, namely, the unilateral cleft of lip and palate, most often seen in males. However, the second most frequent type of cleft, that of the palate only, is predominantly seen in females with a fairly low hereditary background, thus suggesting an entirely different cause.

CLASSIFICATION OF CLEFTS

The incisive foramen seems to serve as a convenient dividing point between the prepalatal clefts (clefts of the primary palate) and the palatal clefts (clefts of the secondary palate). Figure 1-3 shows the three commonest types of palatal clefts.

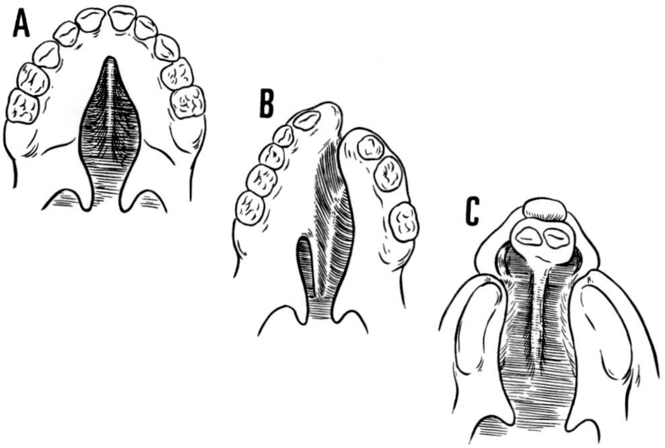

Figure 1-3. The three most common types of palatal clefts. A. Cleft palate only. B. Complete unilateral cleft palate. C. Bilateral cleft palate. Note: B. and C. always involve the lip on the homolateral side.

From L. Bernstein, Congenital Defects of the Oral Cavity. In M.M. Paparella and D.A. Shumrick (Eds.): Otolaryngology, Vol. 111, *Head and Neck,* 1973. Courtsey of W.B. Saunders Company, Philadelphia, Pennsylvania.

Prepalatal Clefts

These may range in extent from a very minor notch in the alveolar process on one side to a complete cleft involving both sides of the anterior palate, alveolar process, lip, and floor of the nasal vestibule (Fig. 1-4A and D). Very rarely, the cleft may be midline, which is considered to be due to lack of fusion of the two median nasal processes.

Palatal Clefts

Midline clefts posterior to the incisive foramen are classified as incomplete and complete and may range from a bifid uvula to a complete cleft extending to the incisive foramen. Included in this classification are the submucous clefts, which may present as a dehiscence of the palatal musculature and/or a cleft in the posterior edge of the bony palate. These are covered with overlying mucous membranes (Fig. 1-4C).

Certain combinations of clefts occur more frequently than

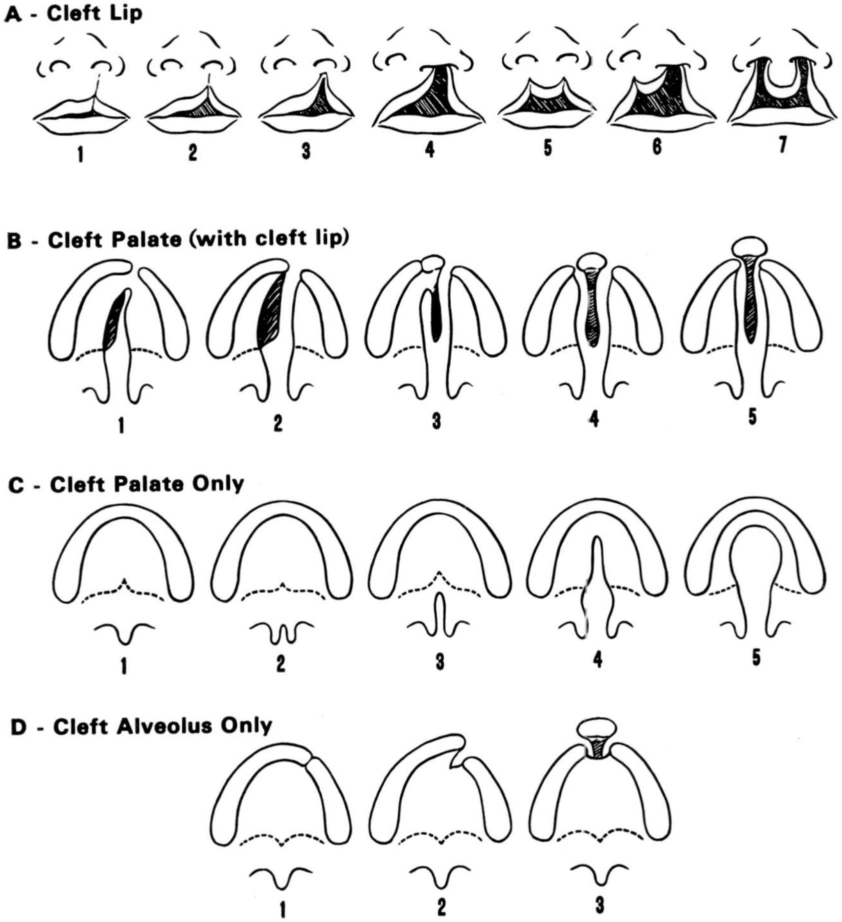

Figure 1-4. A classification of cleft lip and palate based on type, location, and extent.

From L. Bernstein, Congenital Defects of the Oral Cavity. In M.M. Paparella and D.A. Shumrick (Eds.): Otolaryngology, Vol. III, *Head and Neck,* 1973.

Courtesy of W.B. Saunders Company, Philadelphia, Pennsylvania.

others. The most frequent is a left, unilateral, complete cleft of the palate and the prepalatal structures. The second most common is a midline cleft of the soft palate and part of the secondary palate without an accompanying cleft in the prepalatal area.[1] Bilateral clefts of the prepalatal area are usually accompanied by palatal clefts, and incomplete clefts in one area usually accompany incomplete clefts in the other. However, virtually any combination of clefts may occur.

In cases of complete unilateral clefts of the palate and premaxilla, the vomer is attached to the hard palate on the noncleft side; however, when a cleft involves only the secondary palatal structures, the vomer is usually not attached to the maxilla on either side in the region of the cleft.

Other congenital deformities associated with clefts of the palate usually include a very strong predilection to nonsuppurative otitis media, even after the velum has been reconstituted, occasional ankyloglossia and, rarely, pits of the lower lip. Also, in clefts of the secondary palate, the mandible may be underdeveloped, resulting in respiratory embarrassment due to backward displacement of the relatively large tongue. This condition of glossoptosis, micrognathia, and cleft or high-arched palate is commonly referred to as the Pierre Robin syndrome.

REFERENCES

1. Bernstein, L.: The effect of timing of cleft palate operations on subsequent growth of the maxilla. *Laryngoscope, 78:*1510, 1968.
2. Calnan, J.: Modern views on Passavant's ridge. *Br J Plast Surg, 10:*89, 1958.
3. Last, R.J.: *Anatomy: Regional and Applied,* 4th ed. London, J. & A. Churchill Ltd., 1966.
4. Stark, R.B.: Pathogenesis of harelip and cleft palate. *Plast Reconstr Surg, 13:*20, 1954.
5. Walker, B.E.: The association of mucopolysaccharides with morphogenesis of the palate and other structures in mouse embryos. *J Embryol Exp Morphol, 9:*22, 1961.

—2—

EUSTACHIAN TUBE ANATOMY AND PHYSIOLOGY IN THE CLEFT PALATE INDIVIDUAL

Ralph A. Nelson, M.D.

Introduction

THE HUMAN AUDITORY SYSTEM requires an air-containing cavity behind an intact tympanic membrane for its middle ear conductive mechanism to properly function. Sterile, warmed, humified air is transported from the nasopharynx to the tympanic cavity via the eustachian, or auditory, tube. If the eustachian tube becomes obstructed, as in the cleft palate patient, air will not enter the tympanic cavity, and middle ear disease may occur.

Embryology

During the first three weeks of head and neck embryologic development, an endodermal evagination occurs deep in the first pharyngeal pouch separating the first (Meckel's) and second (Reichart's) pharyngeal arches. By the seventh week, this primitive auditory tube migrates laterally through undifferentiated mesenchyme between the two arches to briefly contact ectoderm of the first branchial groove at the site of the future tympanic membrane.

In the third month, growth of second arch mesoderm separates the original evagination into a medial auditory tube and lateral tympanic cavity. The fourth through seventh months represent a time of maturation during which four centers of mesodermal chondrification occur. A more definitive isthmus forms medially, in the fifth month, and a lateral osseous growth further differentiates the auditory tube and tympanic cavity in the sixth and seventh months.

Anatomy

The eustachian tube is an "hourglass" 36 to 37 mm long, connecting the middle ear with the nasopharynx at an angle running lateral to medial, superior to inferior, and posterior to anterior. Generally the tube is at 45° to the saggital plane and 30 to 40° to the horizontal plane. The lateral one-third is osseous and connects with the medial cartilaginous portion at an angle of 160°. The soft tissue two-thirds is at a slightly steeper angulation than the lateral portion. The pharyngeal orifice is 15 mm lower than the tympanic orifice in the adult, but somewhat less in children. At its medial end, the auditory tube mechanism must pass through the sinus of Morgagni where the crescenteric superior constrictor muscle falls short of the skull base (Fig. 2-1). This is immediately opposite the middle of the medial pterygoid plate. In most of its extent, the eustachian tube lies in the petrosphenoidal sulcus

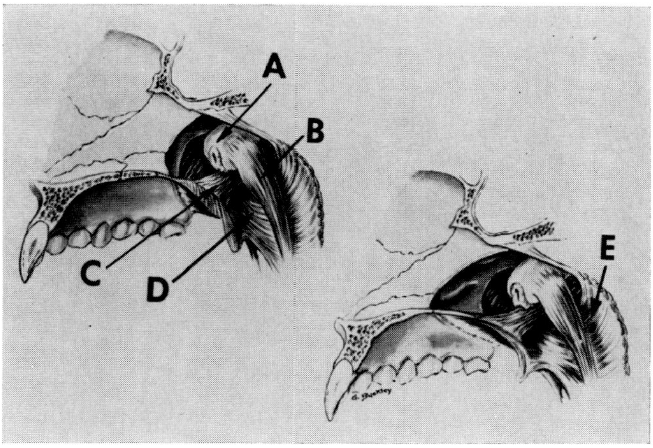

Figure 2-1. The sinus of Morgagni. A. Eustachian tube cartilage. B. Salpingopharyngeus muscle. C. Levator palati. D. Superior constrictor. E. The sinus of Morgagni.

between the petrous apex posteriorly and the greater wing of the sphenoid anteriorly.

Osseous Tube

The bony eustachian tube, approximately 12 mm in length, remains open at all times due to its inflexible wall. Opening into the anterior wall of the tympanic cavity, the tympanic orifice is 5 mm high, 2 mm wide, and progressively narrows as it descends anteriorly. This is largely dependent on its medial and inferior relationship — the carotid canal which is separated from the tube by a thin and sometimes dehiscent bony septum. Its medial roof is the septum canalis musculotubare, which isolates the tensor tympani muscle from the eustachian tube lumen. The middle fossa completes the superior relationship. Laterally, the tympanic part of the temporal bone makes up the wall in a plane parallel to the external auditory canal. Pneumatization surrounding the bony tube may be extensive and provide access to the petrous apex, anterior to the cochlea. Funnel-shaped, the bony tube narrows to 2 mm high and 1 mm wide at the jagged isthmus forming at the junction of the squamous and petrous portions of the temporal bone.

Cartilaginous Tube

Constituting two thirds of the entire length, the soft tissue portion lies in the petrosphenoid sulcus and is composed of a posterior-superior wall of cartilage and an anterior wall of fibroelastic tissue. This portion of the auditory tube, triangular in cross section, is closed at rest (Fig. 2-2). Posteriorly, the wall is a triangular piece of cartilage with its apex inserted into the edge of the bony tube at the isthmus and its base extended into the nasopharynx as the torus tubarius (Fig. 2-3). The cartilage is thin at its lateral insertion, but several mm thick at the torus. In the nasopharynx, the torus represents the posterior wall of the eustachian tube orifice with a superior salpingopalatine ligament extending anteriorly and an inferior fold, the salpingopharyngeus, containing a few slips of muscle which insert into the pharyngeal wall. The slitlike orifice is 9 mm high by 5 mm wide and is separated from the posteriorly located pharyngeal recess (Rosenmüller's fossa) by the torus. The fossa into which the torus is retracted is a pocket measuring 8 to 22 mm deep and 3 to 10 mm wide. Superiorly, a curved domelike edge of the posterior cartilage wall becomes the convex roof of the tube. The extension of the posterior cartilage on cross section completes the short arm of a hook with its anterior side open. A fibroelastic membrane spans the open area between the long and short arms of the hook and forms the anterior-inferior tubal wall (Fig. 2-2). This anterior wall is bounded by the greater wing of the sphenoid superiorly and by the infratemporal fossa inferiorly.

Muscles

The tensor palati is a pretubal muscle originating in the fibrous membrane of the anterior wall (Fig. 2-2). It is thin, flat,

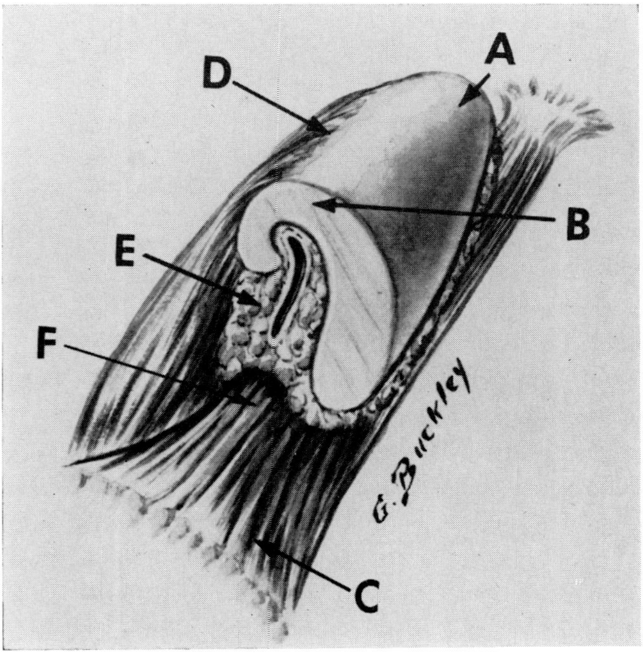

Figure 2-2. Cartilaginous auditory tube. A. Isthmus. B. Cartilage dome. C. Levator palati. D. Tensor palati. E. Ostmann's fat pad. F. Levator palati eminence.

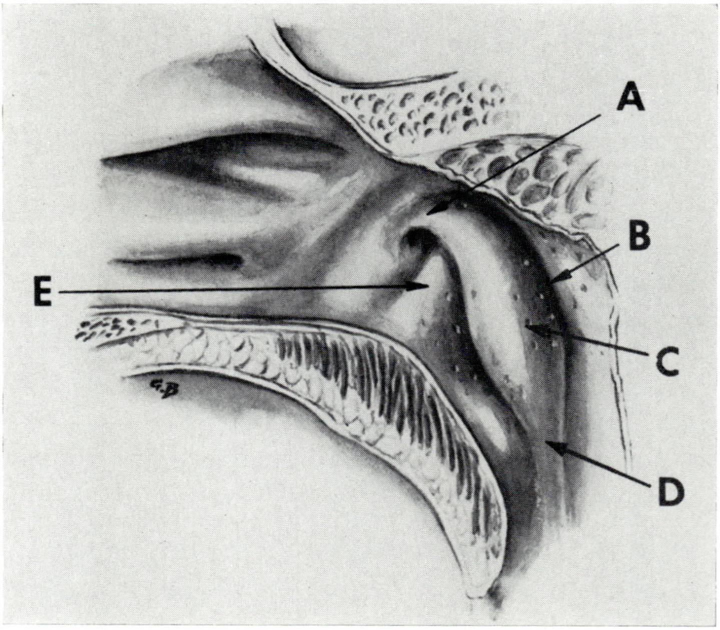

Figure 2-3. Nasopharyngeal ostium of auditory tube. A. Salpingopalatine fold. B. Rosenmeüller's fossa. C. Torus tubarius. D. Salpingopharyngeal fold. E. Levator palati eminence.

triangular, and lies deep in the infratemporal fossa, under the medial pterygoid muscle, the mandibular nerve, and the middle meningeal artery. Arising from the anterior edge of the cartilaginous auditory tube dome, the floor of the scaphoid fossa, and the spine of the sphenoid and the anterior fibroelastic tube, the fibers converge as the muscle descends vertically and perpendicular to the tube between the medial pterygoid plate and medial pterygoid muscle. It ends in a tendon which turns horizontally in a groove on the root of the hamulus. A synovial bursa facilitates movement of the tendon on the hamulus. The muscle then spreads and inserts into the hard palate behind the transverse ridge of the palatal bone and into the aponeurosis of the sofa palate. Innervation of the tensor is the mandibular division of the trigeminal nerve, and vascular supply is by branches of the ascending pharyngeal artery, branches of the internal maxillary artery, the middle meningeal artery, and branches from the ascending palatal artery.

The levator palati muscle occupies a retrotubal position in its origin from the petrous apex anterior to the carotid artery and the posterior cartilaginous wall of the auditory tube (Fig. 2-5). A round, fleshy muscle bundle, it travels parallel to the tube, passing down and forward above the concave margin of the superior constrictor, where it causes a bulge in the floor of the tube and spreads and inserts into the aponeurosis of the dorsal surface of the palate. It is supplied by the branches of the ascending palatine artery and pharyngeal branches of the internal maxillary artery. Innervation is from the bulbar part of the spinal assessory nerve via the pharyngeal plexus.

The salpingopharyngeal muscle is a small structure making up the inferior extension of the torus onto the pharyngeal wall

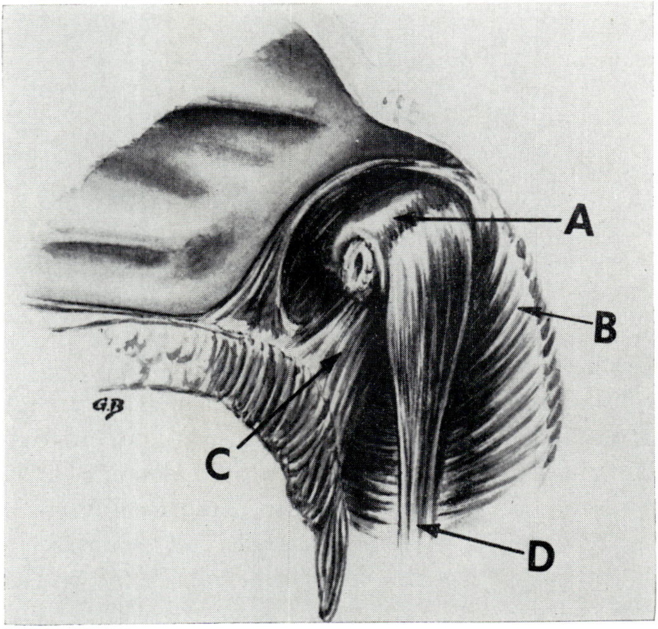

Figure 2-4. Auditory tube muscles. A. Eustachian tube cartilage. B. Superior constrictor. C. Levator palati. D. Salpingopharyngeal muscle.

(Fig. 2-4). Its origin is the torus, and it averages a length of only 4 mm before insertion into the pharyngeal wall. Its vascular supply is the pharyngeal vessels; its innervation is the pharyngeal plexus.

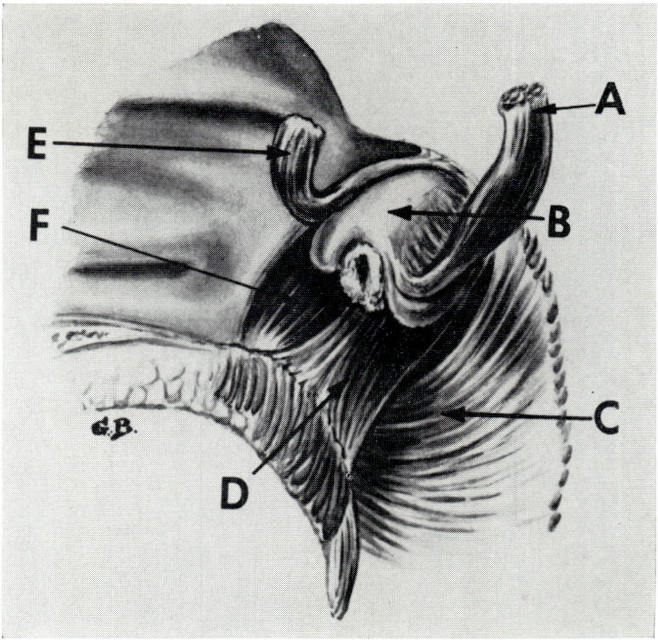

Figure 2-5. Auditory tube muscle. A. Salpingopharyngeal muscle. B. Cartilage dome. C. Superior constrictor. D. Levator palati. E. Cartilage insertion of tensor palati. F. Tensor palati fibroelastic insertion.

The Lumen

The tubal lining is continuous with adjacent structures at each end and, therefore, contains pseudostratified, ciliated columnar epithelium with goblet cells and tubulo alveolar glands at the pharyngeal end before its transition to ciliated columnar epithelium at the tympanic end. A submucosal layer contains lymphatic channels and provides a base for the mucosa. This, in turn, rests on a second, loose layer attached ultimately with a third layer comprising the fibroelastic wall. It is within these layers that Ostmann's fat pad is found.

Vascularity for the tube includes caroticotympanic vessels in the tympanic part, middle meningeal branches in the middle portion, and ascending palatine arteries medially. Sensory innervation of the pharyngeal ostium arises from the pharyngeal plexus' contributions of the glossopharyngeal nerve, while the tympanic end is supplied by Jacobsen's branch of the same nerve. The midportion of the tube is served through the pharyngeal plexus and branches of the greater superficial petrosal nerve.

Venous drainage of the tube and surrounding muscles is through the pericarotid venus plexus, the tympanic veins, and finally the pterygoid plexus. Lymphatic channels in the submucosa drain to parotid nodes through tympanic channels and jugular nodes via retrostyloid and retropharyngeal trunks.

Physiology

At rest, the auditory tube is closed by collapse of the anterior fibroelastic soft tissue wall, by the bulk of Ostmann's fat pad anteriorly, and by the bulk of the fleshy levator palati inferiorly. The tube must be able to open to ventilate the middle ear, release mucous, and equalize pressure differentials created by gaseous absorption and by environmental pressure changes. Opening is provided by muscular action and is probably aided by a surface-active substance diminishing surface tension between opposed mucous membranes.

Muscular action directly dilates the soft part of the tube. All investigators agree that the tensor palati muscle is the most influential muscle of auditory tube opening. However, there is abundant disagreement about the influence, if any, played by the levator palati and other muscles. Whenever a swallow, sneeze, or yawn is initiated, the tensor palati, in addition to tensing the soft palate, also pulls upon the fibroelastic anterior wall and the anterior edge of the cartilage dome. This opens at least the superior two thirds of the lumen, if not the entire channel. Perhaps the levator palati, while elevating the palate, also pulls the posterior wall cartilage and torus into the pharyngeal recess. This muscular action on the lower one third of the lumen may be enhanced by the muscle shortening, with resultant elevation of the tubal floor and lessened opening resistance. The extent of the influence on opening by the salpingopharyngius is unknown.

Normal middle ear pressure is generally accepted as zero, although up to 4 mm Hg negative pressure can be sustained over long periods without evidence of pathologic change. The pressure differential leading to tubal opening has been determined to be 20 to 40 mm. Equalization occurs during the short 0.3 second that the pharyngeal orifice is open.

Since oxygen is more readily absorbed than nitrogen by the mucous membrane of the middle ear, any sustained tubal blockage will result in a negative pressure. Theoretically, the partial pressure of oxygen will decrease from 105 mm in humidified air to that of the surrounding mucous membrane vascular bed (65 mm). If opening fails to take place, tympanic membrane retraction will occur during sustained negative pressure. Multiple theories have evolved to explain fluid accumulation: The most popular is that a transudate from the mucous membrane replaces negative pressure. Recent studies support the hypothesis that negative pressure induces mucosal edema and contributes to mechanical tubal blockage. Another opinion is that infection causes membrane edema and a resulting overproduction of viscous mucus. Radiologic contrast studies have shown that children with middle ear disease and normal palates have evidence of mechanical blockage secondary to mucosal edema. However, children with cleft palates have not shown the same manner of blockage, but rather an inability of the nasopharyngeal orifice to open normally.

Role of Cleft Palate in Auditory Tube Function

The high incidence of middle ear disease in cleft palate patients, especially during formative years, leaves no doubt about the importance of the cleft and its effect on tubal physiology. This may be summarized as (1) failure of the direct opening mechanism, (2) failure of the nasopharyngeal seal, (3) increased tubal compliance, and (4) mucosal edema. Failure of direct muscular opening is perhaps the most obvious problem, since without a proper palatal insertion (Fig. 2-6), the palatal muscles have no anchor to pull against and are unable to dilate the tubal ostium and lumen. This mechanical defect has been the basis for criticism directed toward the practice of hamulus fracture in order to gain better closure during palatal repair. Failure of the nasopharyngeal seal allows the ostium of the tube to be bathed in oral contaminants and could contribute to inflammatory edema of the mucosa. Increased tubal compliance, a finding recently documented, indicated that flaccidity of the tube secondary to muscular dysfunction contributes to obstruction. This problem seems to respond to cleft palate repair or to anatomic maturation of the tube. Mucosal edema is perhaps a secondary occurrence after initial malfunction of the auditory tube has created an altered tympanic cavity.

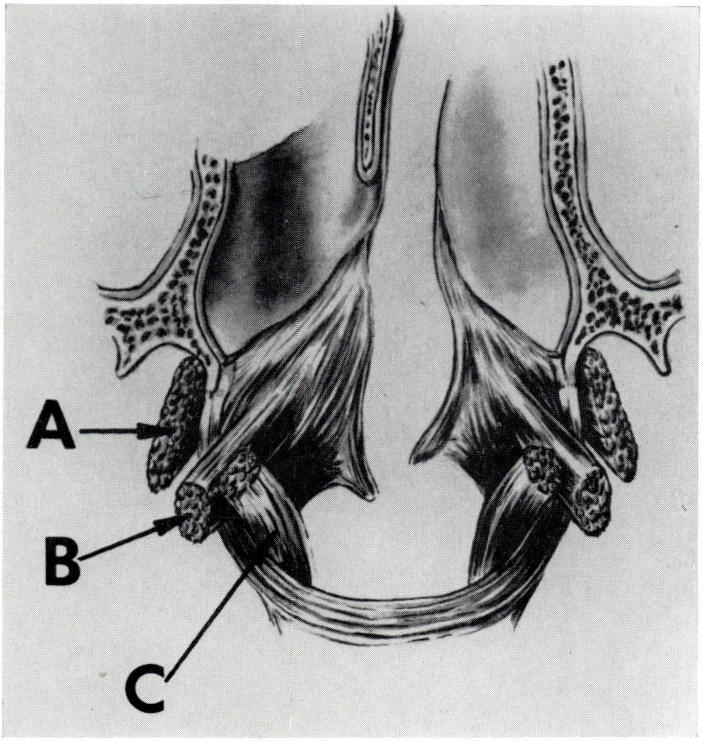

Figure 2-6. Palatal muscle insertions. A. Tensor palati. B. Levator palati. C. Salpingopharyngeal muscle.

The influence of nasopharyngeal adenoid tissue on tubal function in cleft palate patients leads to the question of palatal incompetence if such tissue is removed surgically. If pharyngeal recess obstruction is felt to be adding to tubal dysfunction in the cleft palate child, an adenoidectomy involving only the obstructive tissue of Rosenmüeller's fossa might be considered.

Summary

The normal anatomy and physiology of the eustachian tube has been considered in depth and the abnormal anatomy of the cleft palate discussed. Full knowledge of the concepts presented here is a prerequisite to understanding current thoughts concerning the recognition, diagnosis, and treatment of ear disease in the cleft palate patient.

BIBLIOGRAPHY

Bluestone, C.D.: Eustachian tube obstruction in the infant with cleft palate. *Ann Otol Rhinol Laryngol, 80:*(Suppl 2) 1971.

Brash, J.C.: *Cunningham's Manual of Practical Anatomy, 12th ed.* London, Oxford U Pr, 1958.

Gross, C.M.: *Anatomy of the Human Body,* 27th Ed. Philadelphia, Lea & Febiger, 1959.

Maloney, W.H.: *Otolaryngology.* Hagerstown, Harper & Row, 1973.

Paparella, M.M. and Shumrick, D.A.: *Otolaryngology.* Philadelphia, Saunders, 1973.

Proctor, B.: Embryology and anatomy of the eustachian tube. *Arch Otolaryngol, 86:*51-62, 1967.

Siedentop, K.H., Tardy, M.E., and Hamilton, L.R.: Eustachian Tube Function. *Arch Otolaryngol, 88:*66-75, 1968.

—3—

PREVALENCE AND PATHOGENESIS OF THE EAR DISEASE AND HEARING LOSS

CHARLES D. BLUESTONE, M.D.

Introduction

IN PATIENTS WITH cleft palate, ear disease and hearing loss have long been recognized as common problems. This association was first reported by Alt[1] in 1878, who noted hearing improvement following treatment of otorrhea associated with cleft palate. Thorington[71], in 1892, reported increased hearing in a patient following artificial correction of a destroyed palate. In 1893, Gutzmann[30] noted hearing loss in one half of his patients with cleft palate. Lannois,[38] in 1901, reported the association of middle ear disease and hearing loss in patients with cleft palate. In 1906, the need for otologic examination of patients with cleft palate was stressed by Brunck.[19] Since these early descriptions, many reports have appeared in the literature related to the incidence, nature, and degree of hearing loss in patients with cleft palate.

HEARING LOSS

The prevalence of hearing loss in the cleft palate population, as reported in the literature, varies considerably. The findings of twenty-four recent reports are summarized in Table 3-I. These findings range from 0 percent reported by Goetzinger et al.[27] to

TABLE 3-I.
HEARING LOSS IN CHILDREN AND ADULTS WITH CLEFT PALATE

Investigator	*Year*	*Patients*	*% with Loss*
Sataloff and Fraser[59]	1952	30	90
Means and Irwin[46]	1954	225	59
Holmes and Reed[35]	1955	26	62
Lindsay et al.[39]	1956	390	42
Berry and Eisenson[5]	1956	383	60
Miller[48]	1956	35	54
Halfond and Ballenger[31]	1956	69	75
Whaley[74]	1957	295	25
Pfisterer[56]	1958	54	89
Skolnik[63]	1958	401	39
Linthicum et al.[40]	1959	58	40
Goetzinger et al.[27]	1960	42	0
Drettner[22]	1960	49	63
Masters et al.[43]	1960	172	49
Spriesterbach et al.[66]	1962	163	62
Graham and Lierle[29]	1962	43	51
Graham[28]	1963	190	22
Loeb[41]	1964	108	42
Aschan[3]	1966	82	40
Bennett et al.[7]	1968	30	13
Pannbacher[52]	1969	87	61
Yules[75]	1970	69	58
Bennett[6]	1972	100	58
Walton[73]	1973	93	69

90 percent in the study of Sataloff and Fraser,[59] but of all the studies, the average prevalence is approximately 50 percent. Even though the criteria of hearing loss was not generally agreed upon, it has been identified as conductive and usually bilateral. Halfond and Ballenger[31] found that, of the sixty-nine patients tested, thirty-seven (54%) had a hearing loss of 20 dB or greater. Miller[48] reported that nineteen (54%) of thirty-five children with cleft palate had a hearing loss greater than 30 dB. That the prevalence may be even greater is suggested by Walton,[73] who studied ninety-three school-age children with cleft palate: One half of those who would have passed conventional audiometric screening at the 20 dB level were found to have air-bone gaps indicative of conductive hearing loss. This contention is supported by the study of Bluestone et al.,[13] who found high-viscosity middle ear

effusions in children, including those with cleft palate, who would have passed a 25 dB screening audiogram. Even though a conductive hearing impairment would be expected, Bennett[6] reported 31 percent of 100 adults with cleft palate had either sensorineural or mixed hearing loss. This finding might be explained by the work of Paparella et al.,[53] who found sensorineural hearing loss in some patients with otitis media, and ascribed this to directly associated pathologic changes in the inner ear, presumably mediated via the round window. Unfortunately, no information is available in the literature concerning the hearing in the infant with cleft palate.

AURAL PATHOLOGY

Infants

Variot,[72] in 1904, was the first to report ear disease in an infant with cleft palate. In 1936, Beatty[4] described "acute tubotympanic congestion frequently found between the ages of three months and two years." Sataloff and Fraser,[59] in 1952, reported that, in their experience, "examination of the ears of very young children with cleft palate reveals a high incidence of pathologic changes, despite the absence of subjective symptoms of otitis media." In 1958, Skolnik[63] reported that only 6 percent of cleft palate patients below the age of one, and only 27 percent of those between the ages of one and four years, had aural pathology. Linthicum et al.,[40] however, in 1959, discovered ear pathology in 77 percent of a group of 100 infants and children with cleft palate. In 1967, Stool and Randall[67] reported middle ear effusion was present at myringotomy in 94 percent of twenty-five cleft palate infants. In 1969, Paradise and coworkers,[55] employing standard office otoscopy, diagnosed middle ear disease in forty-nine of fifty infants with cleft palate. Most had full or bulging, opaque, immobile tympanic membranes, although spontaneous perforations and otorrhea were observed. Subsequent studies by the same team indicate that throughout the first two years of life in infants with unrepaired cleft palate, otitis media is a virtually constant complication.[10,54] The otitis is usually characterized by a sterile, inflammatory effusion of variable viscosity; suppuration also occurs occasionally.[10,42,55,65]

Older Children and Adults

Although the criteria of aural pathology in older children and adults with cleft palate varies considerably, its prevalence appears to be quite high. Meissner[47] examined 213 such patients between the ages of ten and thirty-five years and found that 83 percent had abnormal tympanic membranes. Skolnik[63] found the prevalence of aural pathology was 67 percent in patients above the age of five. Graham and Lierle[29] found ear pathology in 44 percent of 29 patients with cleft palate and in 55 percent of 146 with a cleft of both palate and lip. In a group of 82 patients, Aschan[3] found 78 percent had aural pathology. In a retrospective, longitudinal study of 191 patients with cleft palate between five and twenty-seven years of age, Severeid[61] reported 83 percent had a middle ear effusion confirmed by myringotomy. In Bennett's[6] study of 100 adults with cleft palate, 30 percent had aural pathology consisting of signs of eustachian tube obstruction (13%), chronic suppurative otitis media with or without mastoiditis (8%), dry tympanic membrane perforation (6%), and chronic adhesive otitis media (3%).

PATHOGENESIS

Many authors have inferred the pathogenesis of middle ear disease in the patient with cleft palate is the result of eustachian tube dysfunction and, most likely, an obstruction at the nasopharyngeal end.[3,26,32,40,47,49,60,63] Investigation into the exact nature of this dysfunction must be based on the clearest possible understanding of the system constituted by the palate, nasal cavity, nasopharynx, eustachian tube, middle ear, and mastoid air cells. Within this system, the eustachian tube probably has at least three physiologic functions with respect to the middle ear: ventilation, protection from unwanted nasopharyngeal secretions, and drainage of normal or abnormal secretions produced within the middle ear itself. The protective and drainage functions of the eustachian tube in patients with cleft palate have been assessed roentgenographically, utilizing radiopaque media.[10,17] The ventilatory function has been studied by a variety of manometric techniques.[32,33,62] All three functions of the eustachian tube have been studied in infants with cleft palate utilizing both roentgenographic and manometric techniques.[16]

Roentgenographic Studies

Technique

The *protective* function of the eustachian tube can be evaluated by a roentgenographic technique employing radiopaque material instilled through the nose, in order to observe the *retrograde* flow of the medium from the nasopharynx into the eustachian tube.[10,15-18] The technique is as follows.

The patient is restrained, but unanesthetized and unsedated, and placed on the fluoroscopy table in the supine position with the shoulders and trunk elevated on a specially designed holder and the head and neck in posterior extension (Fig. 3-1). This position affords optimal projection for visualization of the nasopharynx-eustachian tube-middle ear-mastoid complex for assessment of retrograde (protective) function of the eustachian tube. A verticosubmental spot roentgenogram is obtained for later comparison. With the subject still in this position, 10 to 20 cc of radiopaque contrast material, sodium diatrizoate 50% weight/volume, is slowly instilled through the nose with a soft rubber catheter under image-intensification fluoroscopic guidance, in order to coat the nasopharynx and to initiate repeated swallowing activity. Retrograde flow of the medium from the nasopharynx into the eustachian tube is observed on the television monitor. This portion of the examination usually only lasts several minutes, since during a very short time, multiple swallows can be observed. The retrograde extent of radiopaque media flow into the eustachian tube is noted during open-nose swallowing. At the completion of this portion of the examination, a second spot roentgenogram is obtained. Following this, the radiopaque material is again instilled while manually closing the nose (roentgenographic Toynbee test). A spot roentgenogram is again obtained. The entire study is permanently recorded on video tape.

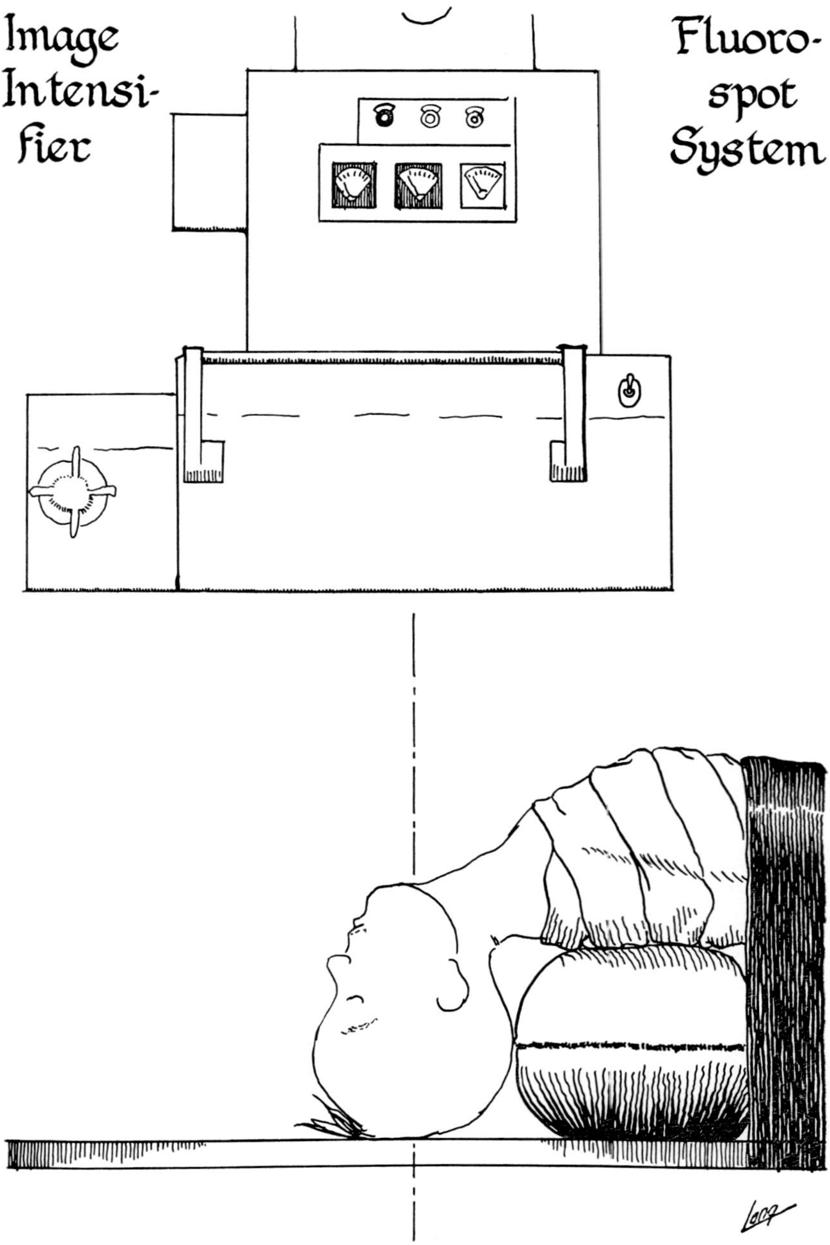

Figure 3-1. Verticosubmental projection employed in roentgenographic assessment of retrograde eustachian tube function.

The retrograde function of the eustachian tube at its nasopharyngeal end can be classified into the following types
1. Normal Retrograde Function—Toynbee Negative: At rest the normal eustachian tube remains functionally closed, with no contrast material entering it. With each open-nose swallow, however, the tube opens, and radiopaque media spurts jetlike into the proximal one third or one half of the tube and then immediately returns. No contrast material enters the middle ear during closed-nose swallowing (Fig. 3-2).

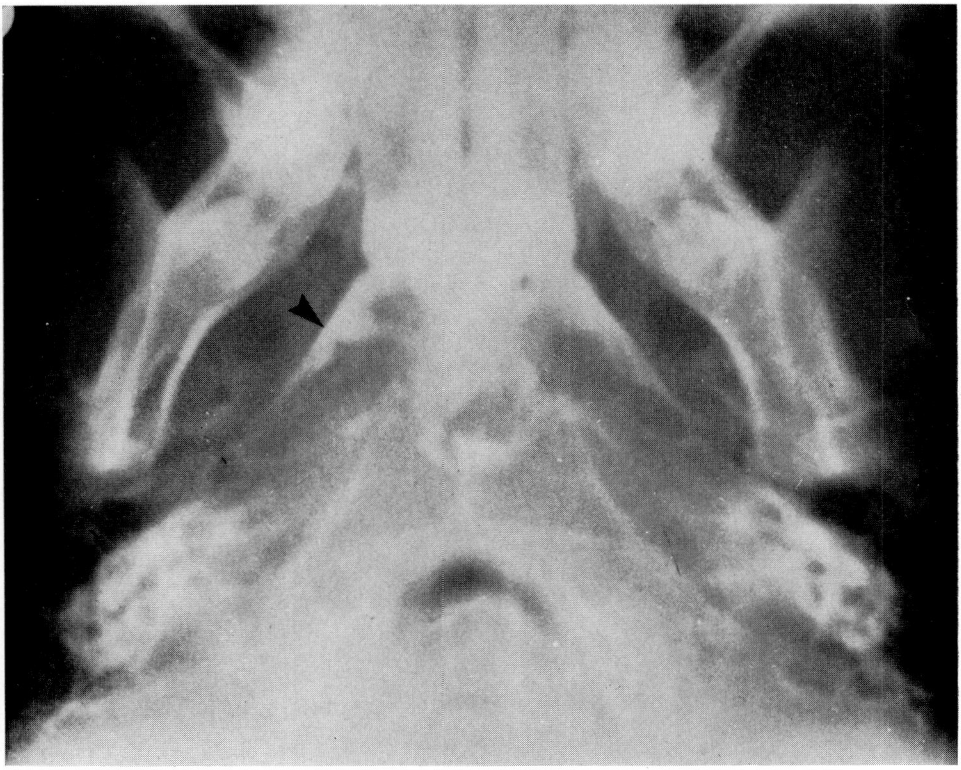

Figure 3-2. Normal retrograde function — Toynbee negative. During open-nose swallowing, radiopaque contrast material filled the nasopharyngeal portion of the eustachian tube (arrow) of a child with normal palate and tympanic membranes. No contrast media entered the middle ear during closed-nose swallowing.

2. NORMAL RETROGRADE FUNCTION—TOYNBEE POSITIVE: During open-nose swallowing, retrograde function appears normal, but when the nares are manually compressed, contrast media traverses the eustachian tube and enters the middle ear (Fig. 3-3).

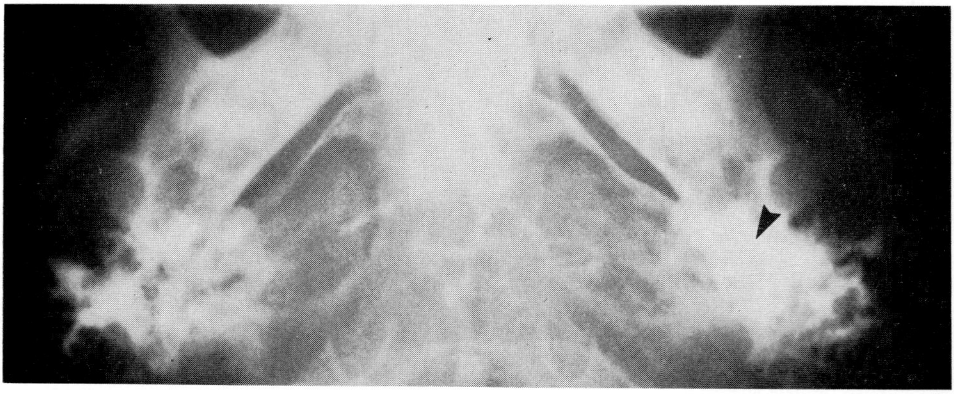

Figure 3-3. Normal retrograde function — Toynbee positive. Roentgenogram of a six-year-old boy with normal palate and otitis media, who had normal retrograde function during open-nose swallowing. During closed-nose swallowing, contrast material traverses the eustachian tube and enters the middle ear and mastoid (arrow).

3. RETROGRADE REFLUX: Upon open-nose swallowing, contrast media traverses the entire length of the eustachian tube and refluxes into the middle ear (Fig. 3-4).
4. RETROGRADE OBSTRUCTION—TOYNBEE POSITIVE: During open-nose swallowing, contrast material fails to enter the nasopharyngeal end of the eustachian tube, but upon closed-nose swallowing, radiopaque media enters the middle ear (Fig. 3-5).
5. RETROGRADE OBSTRUCTION—TOYNBEE NEGATIVE: During both open and closed-nose swallowing, contrast material fails to enter the eustachian tube upon repeated swallowing (Fig. 3-6).

The drainage (clearance) function of the eustachian tube can then be studied by the following technique.

Following completion of the foregoing retrograde study, the patient is turned to the prone position for the *prograde* clearance study. If contrast material has entered the middle ear end of the

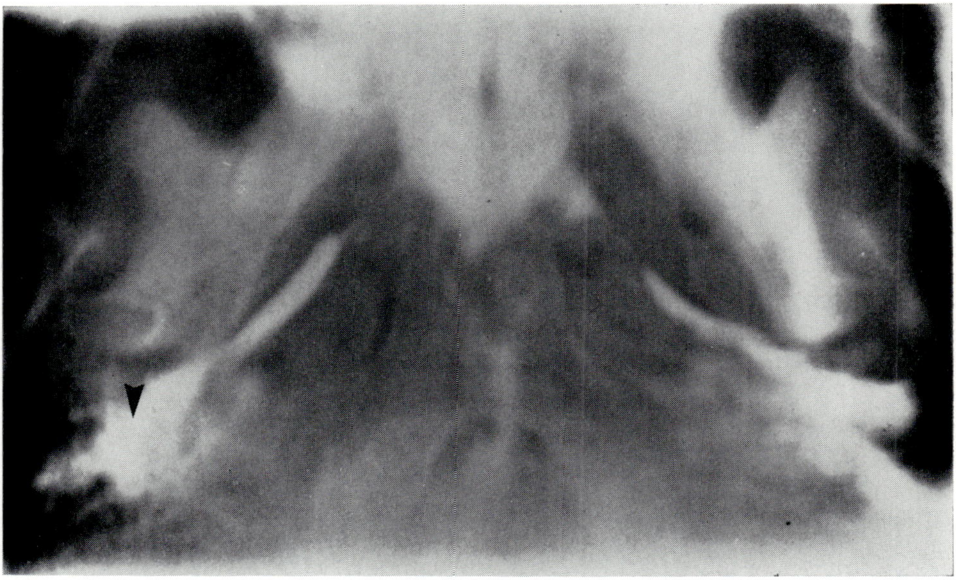

Figure 3-4. Retrograde reflux. Roentgenogram of a six-year-old boy with normal palate and otitis media. Upon open-nose swallowing, contrast material traverses the entire eustachian tube and enters the middle ear and mastoid (arrow).

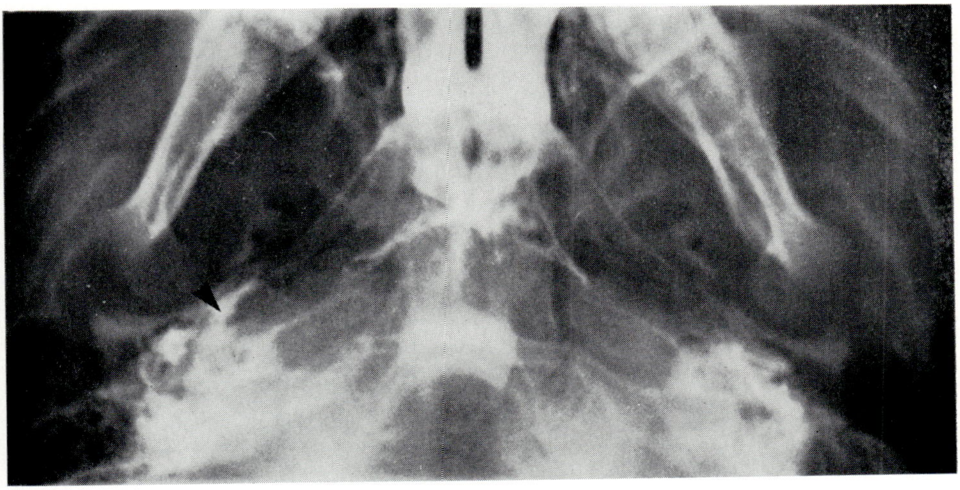

Figure 3-5. Retrograde obstruction – Toynbee positive. Roentgenogram of a four-year-old boy with normal palate and otitis media. During open-nose swallowing, contrast media failed to enter the nasopharyngeal portion of the eustachian tube; however, radiopaque material entered the middle ear and mastoid (arrow) during closed-nose swallowing.

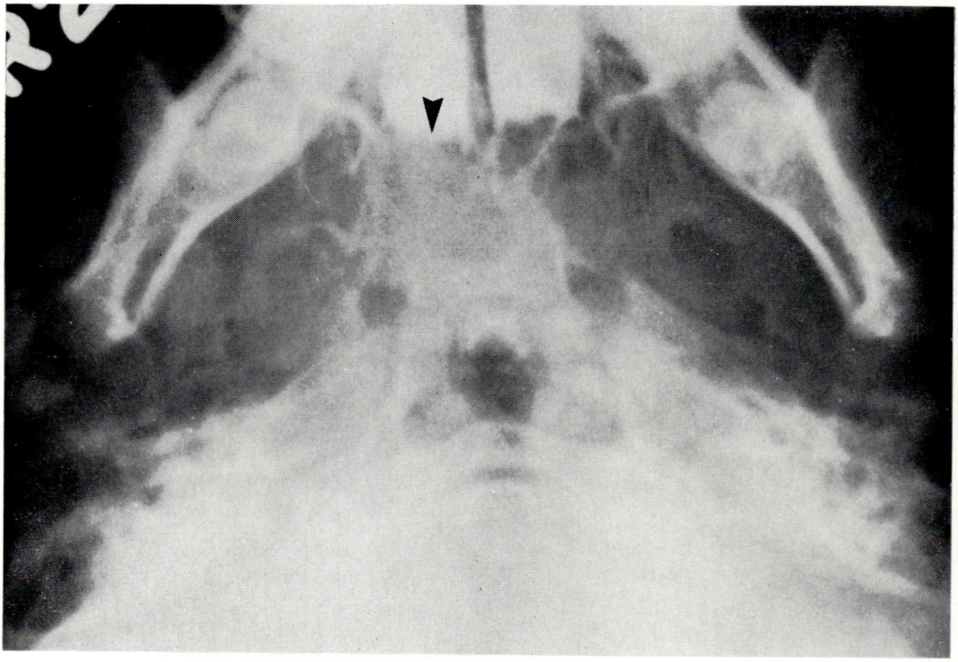

Figure 3-6. Retrograde obstruction — Toynbee negative. Roentgenogram of a five-year-old boy with normal palate and otitis media. Radiopaque media failed to enter the nasopharyngeal portion of the eustachian tube during both open and closed-nose swallowing. Note the enlarged adenoids (arrow).

eustachian tube and the middle ear during the retrograde examination, the patient is kept in the prone position for ten minutes, a final submentovertical spot roentgenogram is obtained, and the degree of clearance of the contrast material from the middle ear is noted.

If contrast material has not previously entered the middle ear, and if a tympanostomy tube or perforation is present, some additional contrast material is instilled through the tube by means of a small-bore needle. The middle ear must be dry and aerated for an accurate assessment of the drainage function. If the material does not clear from the middle ear within ten minutes, or if, on the other hand, it does clear, with good visualization of the middle ear and bony portion of the eustachian tube, the study can be terminated.

In the *prograde* studies, if contrast material clears from the mastoid, middle ear, and bony portion of the eustachian tube into the nasopharynx within ten minutes, clearance is considered satisfactory. If not, and if the middle ear portion of the eustachian tube can be visualized and appears patent, the study is considered to indicate prograde obstruction of the eustachian tube (Fig. 3-7).

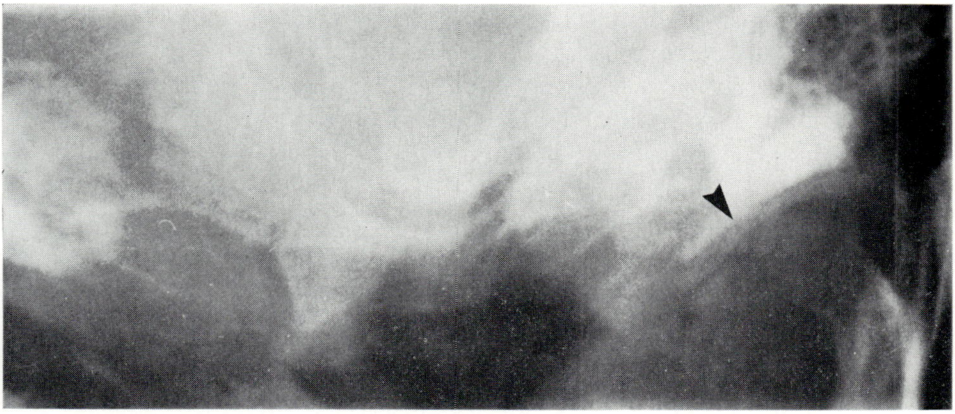

Figure 3-7. Prograde obstruction. Roentgenogram of a six-year-old boy with normal palate and typmpanostomy tube in place. Radiopaque media failed to flow from the bony portion of the eustachian tube (arrow) into the nasopharynx.

Interpretation of Roentgenographic Studies

The eustachian tube is considered to have normal *protective* and *drainage* function when, upon both open and closed-nose swallowing, radiopaque material enters only the nasopharyngeal or isthmus portions of the tube and does not enter the bony portion of the tube or the middle ear cavity (retrograde normal—Toynbee negative). The eustachian tube would appear to protect the middle ear from the low-viscosity contrast material, even when the liquid is under increased pressure. Successful clearance of radiopaque media from the middle ear into the nasopharynx would indicate normal drainage function of the eustachian tube.

If, during the retrograde study, contrast material traverses the entire eustachian tube and enters the middle ear during either open-nose (retrograde reflux) or closed-nose (roentgenographic Toynbee positive) swallowing, the tube is considered to have increased distensibility and probably poor protective function. Failure of the contrast material to drain from the middle ear into the nasopharynx (prograde obstruction) would indicate anatomic or *mechanical* obstruction of the eustachian tube, especially when contrast material also fails to enter the nasopharyngeal portion of the tube during the retrograde study (retrograde obstruction). Mechanical obstruction can either be intrinsic or extrinsic. Prograde obstruction, when associated with normal retrograde function probably indicates mechanical obstruction within the isthmus portion of the eustachian tube.

Studies in Infants with Unrepaired Cleft Palate

Roentgenographic studies of infants with unrepaired cleft palate employing the technique previously described, showed that all have *retrograde obstruction* to the flow of liquid contrast material into the nasopharyngeal portion of the eustachian tube during both open and closed- nose swallowing (Fig. 3-8). Normal function has not been observed.[10,16,17]

Prograde clearance was demonstrated to some degree in all ears; however, the degree of clearance of the material varied with both viscosity and the position of the patient. In many ears, high-viscosity media and the supine position were associated with incomplete clearance of the media from the middle ear and mastoid and, in a few infants, clearance appeared to depend on the presence of a functioning tympanostomy tube.

Studies in Infants and Young Children with Repaired Cleft Palate

The protective and drainage function of the eustachian tube were studied in infants with cleft palate, both before and after surgical repair.[16] Following surgical repair of the palate, there was improvement in prograde clearance and, in over one half of the ears tested, retrograde flow appeared normal during open-

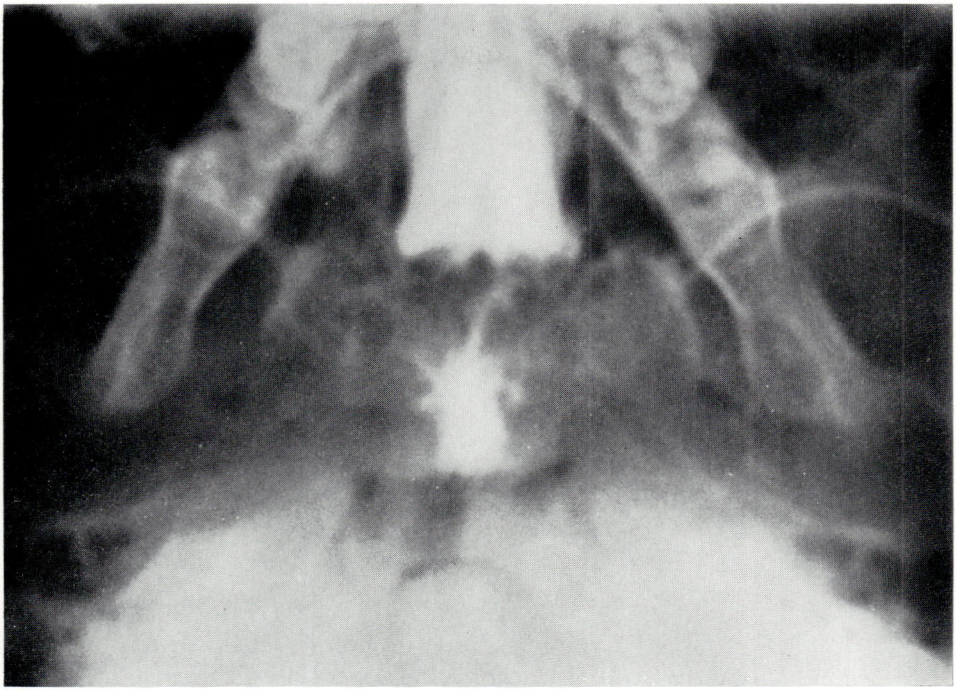

Figure 3-8. Retrograde obstruction in an infant with an unrepaired cleft palate. During both open and closed-nose swallowing, radiopaque contrast material failed to enter the eustachian tube (roentgenographic Toynbee negative).

nose swallowing. Prior to repair of the palate, the *roentgenographic Toynbee test* had been negative in all ears tested. Following repair, however, the test was positive in 86 percent (Fig. 3-9).

Ventilation Studies

Technique

Ventilatory function of the eustachian tube can be studied by a modification of an inflation-deflation technique developed by Flisberg and coworkers.[24] If a tympanostomy tube or perforation is present, the pump-manometer portion of the electro acoustic impedance bridge can be used.[12-16] Figure 3-10 shows the symbols employed and examples of the results obtained in the ventilation

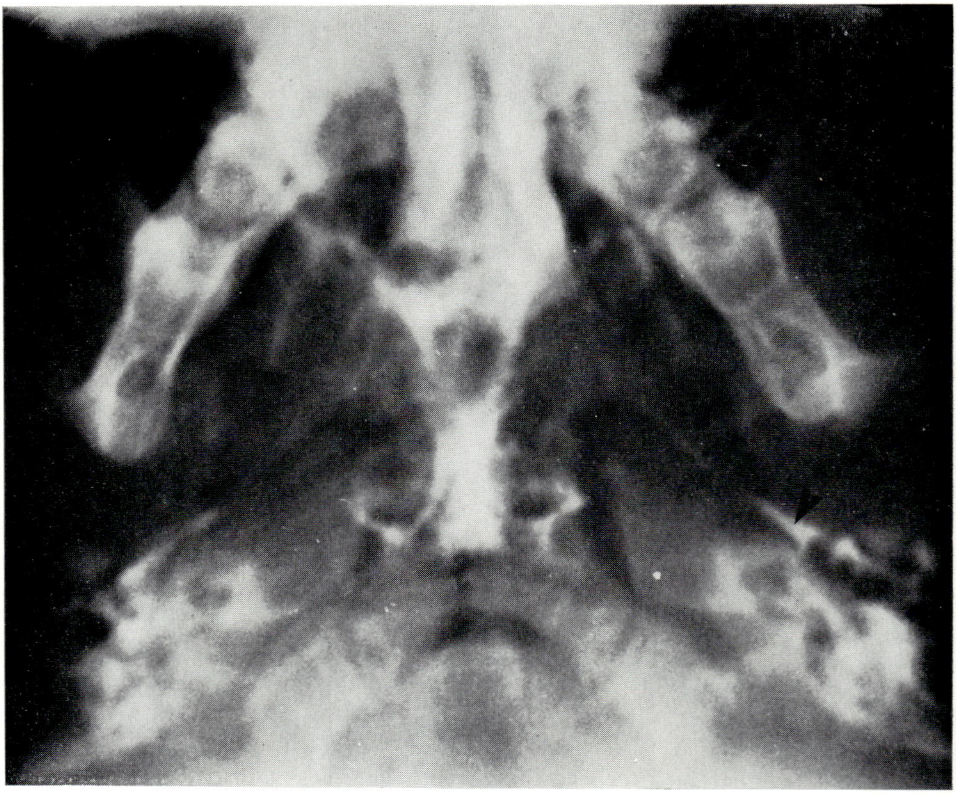

Figure 3-9. Roentgenogram of an infant with a repaired cleft palate demonstrating a "positive roentgenographic Toynbee test." Note the contrast material in the middle ear cavity (arrow).

studies. Example A. describes a study of a normal adult with a traumatic perforation but an otherwise negative otologic history. After sealing the external canal with the probe tip, pressure was applied — *inflation* — until passive opening of the tube occurred. This pressure-induced tubal opening is called the *opening pressure,* and the residual external canal-middle ear pressure, after the tube closes, the *closing pressure.* Active swallowing by the patient completely equilibrated the remaining positive pressure. The external canal-middle ear pressure was then reduced — *de-*

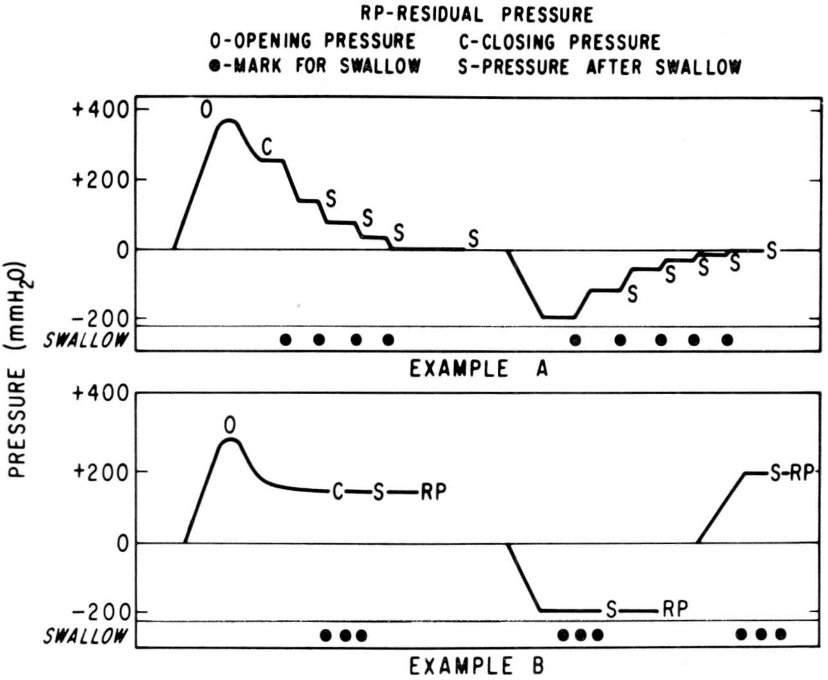

Figure 3-10. Symbols and examples of results during inflation-deflation ventilation studies. Example A. a normal adult with a traumatic perforation of the tympanic membrane but an otherwise negative otologic history. Example B. a four-year-old patient with a repaired cleft palate and a functioning tympanostomy tube in the test ear.

flation — to —200 mm H_2O. This negative pressure was also completely equilibrated by the patient's swallowing activity. Example B. describes a study of a four-year-old patient with a repaired cleft palate. The test ear had a functioning tympanostomy tube in place. The eustachian tube passively opened and closed following inflation, but subsequent swallowing failed to equilibrate the *residual positive pressure.* In the deflation phase of the study, the child was unable to equilibrate negative pressure. Inflation to a pressure below the opening pressure but above the closing pressure could not be equilibrated by active swallow function.

Studies in Patients with Traumatic Perforations of the Tympanic Membrane

Figure 3-11 is a summary of the inflation-deflation ventilation studies of twenty-four patients (twenty-four ears) with normal palate, traumatic perforation of the tympanic membrane, but an otherwise negative otologic history. Their ages ranged from two to fifty-two years. The ages of the only five children in the group are identified in the figure. In all twenty-four ears, the eustachian tube opened at or below applied middle ear pressure equal to

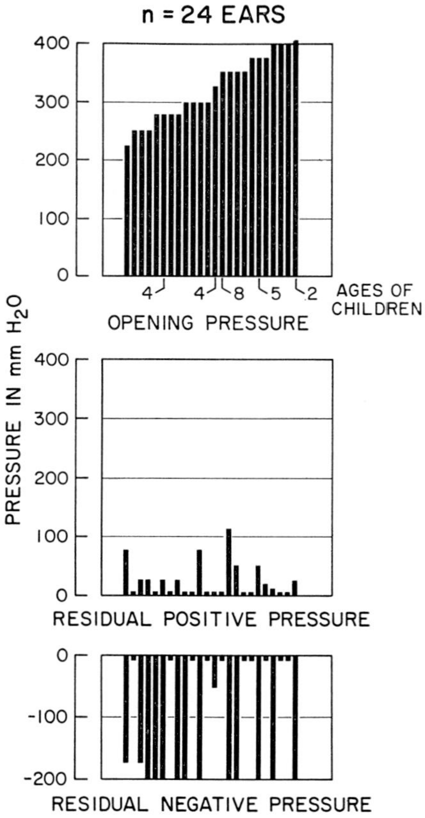

Figure 3-11. Ventilation studies of twenty-four patients (twenty-four ears) with normal palates and with traumatic perforations of the tympanic membrane, but otherwise negative otologic histories.

+410 mm H_2O. Twenty-three ears (96%) had residual positive air pressure below +100 mm H_2O, while in only one ear the residual positive pressure was 120 mm H_2O. Ten of the twenty-four ears tested (42%) were able to completely equilibrate applied negative pressure. In three ears (12%) negative pressure was partially equilibrated, while in eleven ears (46%) negative pressure could not be equilibrated at all.

Even though a variety of eustachian tube responses were obtained, it must be assumed that these ventilatory function tests are within normal limits. However, almost one half of the subjects in this group were unable to equilibrate applied negative middle ear pressure by swallowing. This response, when associated with low opening pressure, would suggest a tube with less stiffness (increased compliance) than one through which both negative and positive pressures could be completely equilibrated. Most likely these eustachian tubes were temporarily locked during the negative phase of the test.

Studies in Infants with Unrepaired Cleft Palate

Twenty-one infants with unrepaired cleft palate had eustachian tube ventilation studies in thirty-two ears that were intubated (tympanostomy tube), aerated, and dry.[14] Figure 3-12 shows the results of these studies. Figure 3-12 (upper frame) shows that, in nine ears (28%), the eustachian tube opened (solid line) at or below a positive middle ear pressure equal to +400 mm H_2O, whereas in twenty-three ears (72%), the eustachian tube did not open (broken line) in response to the applied positive middle ear pressure equal to +400 mm H_2O. (These eustachian tubes might have opened if a greater positive pressure had been applied; however, this was not possible due to the limitations of the instrument.) Figure 3-12 (middle frame) shows that, in thirty ears (94%), residual pressure greater than +100 mm H_2O remained in the middle ear following either pressure-induced opening of the eustachian tube, swallowing, or both. Figure 3-12 (lower frame) shows that none of the subjects tested was able to equilibrate negative middle ear air pressure equal to –200 mm H_2O by swallowing.

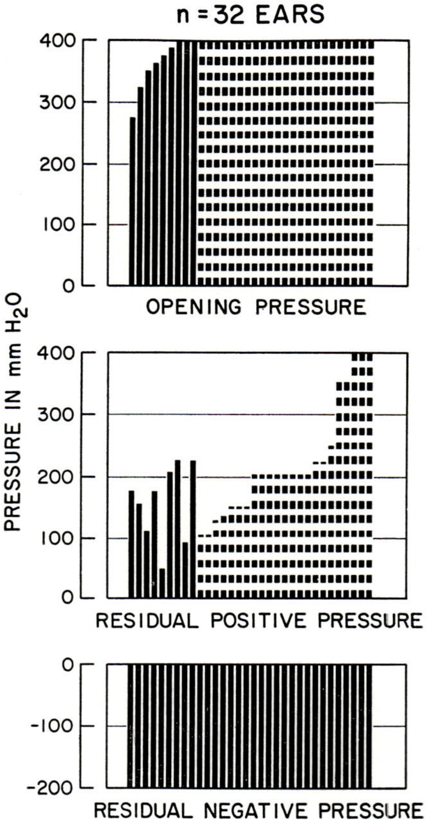

Figure 3-12. Ventilation studies of twenty-one infants with unrepaired cleft palate in thirty-two ears that were intubated, aerated, and dry.

Studies in Infants and Children with Repaired Cleft Palate

Figure 3-13 shows the inflation-deflation studies obtained on fifty-eight ears of the thirty-seven infants and children with repaired palatal clefts. In forty-seven ears (81%), the eustachian tube opened (solid line) at or below a positive pressure equal to +400 mm H_2O, whereas in only eleven ears (19%) did the eustachian tube fail to open (broken line) in response to applied positive pressure equal to +400 mm H_2O. In twenty-six ears (45%), residual positive pressure greater than +100 mm H_2O

remained in the middle ear after the attempt to equilibrate by swallowing. None of these subjects was able to equilibrate applied negative middle ear pressure.

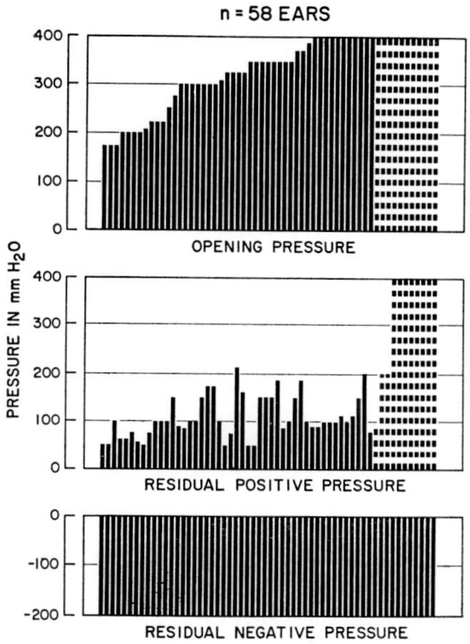

Figure 3-13. Ventilation studies of thirty-seven infants and children with repaired cleft palate in fifty-eight ears that were intubated, aerated, and dry.

Cleft Palate and Eustachian Tube Obstruction

These liquid and air-flow studies indicate that infants with unrepaired cleft palates are conditionally able to clear radiopaque liquid media from the middle ear and eustachian tube into the nasopharynx, but there is obstruction to retrograde flow from the nasopharynx into the eustachian tube. Such infants also appear to have a variable degree of difficulty equilibrating increased middle ear pressure and are unable to equilibrate negative pressure by active function (swallowing). The presence of high residual positive pressures during the inflation phase of the test would indicate some degree of obstruction to air flow through the eustachian tube. It appears likely that their tubes are abnormally compliant, so that during swallowing, the pull of the tensor veli palatini muscle may be inadequate to produce effective tubal opening. The eustachian tube appears to be less obstructed in patients whose palates have been repaired, since those patients have lower opening pressures and lower residual positive pressures, and since they show improvement in the flow of liquid contrast media through the eustachian tube in both retrograde and prograde directions.

It would appear that the eustachian tube of children with cleft palate, both before and after repair, may lack stiffness or have increased compliance. Collapse of such a tube might then result in functional tubal obstruction. If this is so, the tube would be persistently collapsed even during swallowing, and a greater than normal pressure differential between the nasophraynx and the middle ear would be required to open the tube and accomplish middle ear ventilation. In support of this concept are (1) the frequent finding of tympanic membrane retraction and (2) tympanometric evidence of negative middle ear pressure in many children with cleft palates.[8,16]

In infants with unrepaired cleft palate, therefore, the sequence of events is probably as follows: initially, negative pressure is present in the middle ear as a result of *functional obstruction* of the eustachian tube and constant absorption of gas within the middle ear cavity. A middle ear effusion results. Aschan[2] found edema, hyperemia, diapedesis of leukocytes, and transudation in the middle ear mucous membrane of rabbits subjected to hypoxia. Flisberg et al.,[25] utilizing a percutaneous cannula in the mastoid process in normal subjects, found a middle ear effusion after 15 minutes of the application of –20 to –30 mm of mercury. Once a middle ear effusion is present, persistent negative middle ear pressure, secondary to functional obstruction of the eustachian tube, could prevent drainage. Negative middle ear pressure and decreased oxygen would also have a deleterious effect on the mucociliary transport system and result in an increase in mucus-secreting cells.[58] Mucosal swelling in the middle ear end of the eustachian tube, increased quantity and viscosity of the effusion, adhesion of the liquid to the bony walls of the cavity, and surface tension of the liquid could also prevent successful clearance of the middle ear cavity.[10,12] The finding of relatively asymptomatic, sterile middle ear effusion in infants with unrepaired cleft palates would tend to support these hypothetical considerations.

In an effort to eliminate the middle ear effusion in the infant with an unrepaired cleft palate, tympanostomy tubes have been advocated.[10,21] The success of the tympanostomy tube is most likely related to the prevention of negative middle ear pressure and hypoxia and improvement in drainage of mucus from the middle ear into the nasopharynx. However, otorrhea through the tympanostomy tubes has been the chief otic complication.[10,54] The presence of a perforation of the tympanic membrane or a tympanostomy tube could permit nasopharyngeal secretions to enter the middle ear, since the eustachian tube is only functionally obstructed, and the middle ear and mastoid air cells no longer constitute a closed compartment.[11] Accessibility of nasopharyngeal secretions at the mouth of the eustachian tube would be enhanced by the supine body position.

Effect of Palate Repair on Eustachian Tube Function and Middle Ear Status

Following repair of the cleft palate, the same mechanisms responsible for middle ear effusions in the infant prior to surgical correction of the palate would be operative if functional obstruction of the eustachian tube persists. However, many children with repaired cleft palate are subject to occurrences of acute media. Increased distensibility of the eustachian tube, as well as successful velopharyngeal closure following surgical correction of the cleft, may be related to this observation. Closed-nose swallowing, when the palate is intact and the velopharyngeal valving mechanism competent, could result in either a monophasic positive or negative pressure excursion or a biphasic positive-negative excursion in the nasopharynx.[36] Nasal obstruction can occur with inflammation. The effect of these pressures on a pliant tube could result in the *Toynbee phenomenon*,[12,16] as described below. During the positive phase, nasopharyngeal secretions might be forced into the middle ear, especially when the middle ear has high negative pressure. During the negative phase, such a tube easily could be locked (Fig. 3-14). High negative middle ear pressure, even when the nose is not obstructed, would result in a large nasopharyngeal-middle ear pressure gradient. If ventilation occurs, and the tube is sufficiently distensible, nasopharyngeal secretions might be aspirated into the middle ear. This could readily occur in a pliant tube, even with high-viscosity nasopharyngeal secretions, and could result in acute bacterial otitis media.

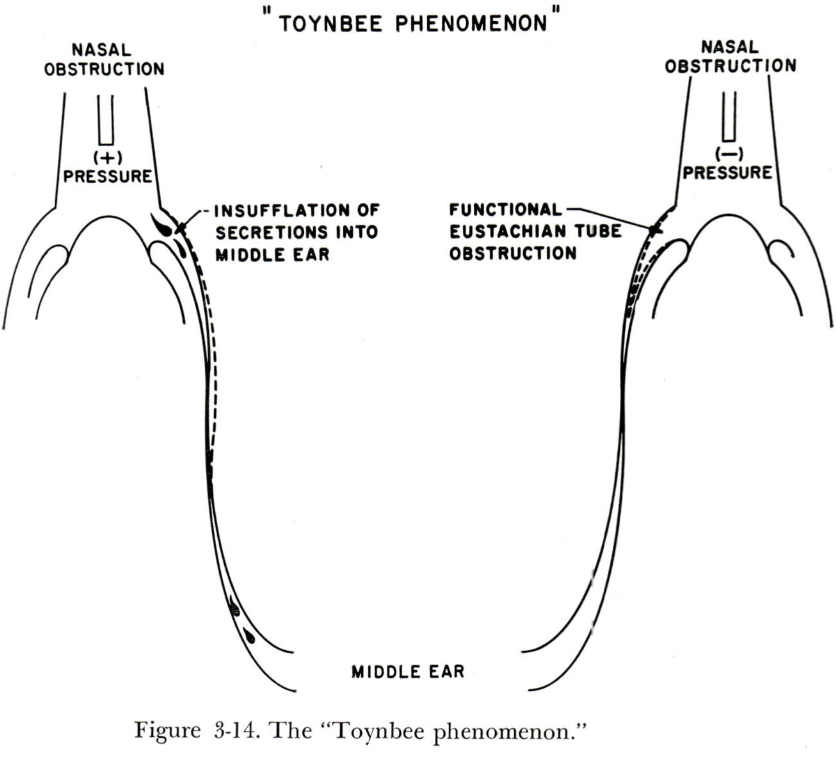

Figure 3-14. The "Toynbee phenomenon."

Palate repair, however, appears to result in a sharp improvement in middle ear status.[3,43,56,65] Bluestone et al.[16] studied the eustachian tube function and examined the ears of infants with cleft palate, both before and after repair of the posterior palate.

Prior to repair, middle ear effusion was uniformly present. Six to twelve months following repair, one half were free of disease. The improvement in otologic status was attributed to improvement in eustachian tube function. In a later study, Paradise and Bluestone[54] studied ninety-two infants with cleft palate, both before and after surgical correction of the palate. The otologic status was related to the need for myringotomy and tympanostomy tube insertion. An overall reduction in frequency of myringotomy following repair was found, which was not attributed merely to the fact that the children had grown older.

Improvement of middle ear status following repair of the cleft palate may be related to the observed increase in the distensibility of the eustachian tube. Achievement of velopharyngeal closure may also improve middle ear ventilation, possibly related to improvement in the tensor veli palatini muscle tension or vector. Following successful palate repair, periodic nasal obstruction could "pump" air into the middle ear cavity during closed-nose swallowing, conpensating for persistent functional eustachian tube obstruction. Naturally, this mechanism would not be operative prior to palate repair.

Pterygold Hamulotomy and Eustachian Tube Function

The technique of pterygoid hamulotomy has been widely utilized during the repair of the cleft palate, in an effort to reduce the tension placed on the muscle sling.[9] This practice has been related to the occurrence of otitis media by some investigators,[26,32,33,57,63] while others have reported no increased incidence following the procedure.[7,16] Following unilateral hamulotomy in animals, Odoi et al.[51] reported the development of middle ear effusion. They, however, "expunged" the hamulus in these animals. Thompson and Harwood-Nash[70] studied the fate of the infractured hamuli in five infants both before and after palate repair. By using a wire sutured to the hamulus, they found the hamulus returned to its preoperative position following infracture. Bluestone et al.[16] reported that unilateral hamulotomy undertaken during the course of cleft palate repair appeared to have no effect on either eustachian tube function or the recurrence of middle ear effusions. These findings are in agreement with those of Noone et al.[50] in a larger series of patients.

Age, Eustachian Tube Function, and Middle Ear Status

The incidence of otitis media in the child with cleft palate, as well as in those with normal palates, progressively decreases with advancing age.[61] This may be related to increase in cartilage support of the eustachian tube or the muscle vectors, which may improve with the craniofacial growth and development occurring at puberty. From air-pressure and liquid-flow studies, even some children with normal palates and a negative otologic history have eustachian tubes that are more compliant or have inefficient active opening mechanisms, as compared to adults. Holborow[33] has studied the cross-sectional increase in the Eustachian tube cartilage in the older child, as compared with the infant. Ross[57] examined the muscle vectors of the tensor veli palatini and found a difference in the child as compared with the adult. However, the eustachian tube of the child with cleft palate appears to have worse function than the child with a normal palate. Subtenly[68] reported that the bihamular measurements and the nasopharynx in general are wider in young children with cleft palate as compared with subjects who had normal palates. This variation could alter the vectors of the tensor veli palatini muscle. In 1969, Surina and Jagr[69] reported their electromyographic study of patients with cleft palate and concluded that the action potentials they observed, as well as histologic evidence they collected, demonstrated reduced contractile tissue and increased connective tissue in the tensor and levator muscles. Kriens[37] and Fara and Dvorok[23] found the tensor veli palatini muscle hypoplastic in autopsies of unoperated cleft newborns. Dickson[20] studied cleft palate and noncleft human fetuses to determine whether differences in the eustachian tube and cranial base structures could be found which would explain the universal appearance of middle ear effusion in infants with cleft palate. Principal findings included medial to lateral compression of the eustachian tube and reduced tube width. These findings could reduce eustachian tube stiffness.

Implications

Since middle ear disease in patients with cleft palate appears to result from functional eustachian tube obstruction, which can result in negative middle ear pressure, it seems reasonable to maintain normal middle ear pressure. This can usually be accomplished by the insertion of tympanostomy tubes.[10,54] The overall reduction in middle ear disease following palate repair would appear to constitute a basis for considering earlier repair than might otherwise by undertaken.[54] Paradise et al.[35] have pointed out that the middle ear damage and hearing loss prevalent during later life in patients with cleft palate probably originates with chronic middle ear effusion in infancy, and they have suggested further that the restrictions of language skill[45] and psychological problems[44,64] seemingly prevalent in later life may have the same origin, since the persistent middle ear effusion of infants with cleft palate is probably accompanied by variable degrees of hearing loss. Holm and Kunze[34] found significantly retarded language development in school-age children without cleft palate but with persistent middle ear disease. The risk in later life by infants with cleft palate would appear to justify early and prolonged treatment of their middle ear effusions.

REFERENCES

1. Alt. A.: Heilunger Taubstummheit erzielte durch beseitigung einer Otorrhoe und einer angebornen Gaumenspalte. *Arch für Augen und Ohrenh, 7:*211, 1878; and *Schmidt's Jahrbuecher, 183:*277, 1879.
2. Aschan, G.: Aero-otitis media and aero-sinusitis. *Acta Otolaryngol,* Suppl 69, 1948.
3. Aschan, G.: Hearing and nasal function correlated to postoperative speech in cleft palate patients with velopharyngoplasty. *Acta Otolaryngol, 61:*371-379, 1966.
4. Beatty, H.G.: The care of cleft palate patients. *Laryngoscope, 46:*203, 1936.
5. Berry, M.F. and Eisenson, J.: *Speech Disorders: Principles and Practices of Therapy.* New York, Appleton-Century-Crofts Inc., 1956.
6. Bennett, M.: The older cleft palate patient. *Laryngoscope, 82:*1217-1225, 1972.
7. Bennett, M., Ward, R.H. and Tait, C.A.: Otologic-audiologic study of cleft palate children. *Laryngoscope, 78:*1011-1019, 1968.
8. Bess, F.H., Lewis, H.D., and Cieliczka, D.J.: Acoustic impedance mea-

surements in cleft palate children. *J Speech Hear Disord, 40:*13-24, 1975.

9. Bilroth, T.: Ueber uranoplastik. *Wien Klin Wochenschr, 2:*241, 1889.
10. Bluestone, C.D.: Eustachian tube obstruction in the infant with cleft palate. *Ann Otol Rhinol Laryngol* [Suppl 2], *80:*1-30, 1971.
11. Bluestone, C.D. and Berry, Q.C.: Concepts in the pathogenesis of middle ear effusions. *Ann Otol Rhinol Laryngol* [Suppl 25], *85:*182-186, 1976.
12. Bluestone, C.D., Beery, Q.C., and Andrus, W.S.: Mechanics of the Eustachian tube as it influences susceptibility to and persistence of middle ear effusions in children. *Ann Otol Rhinol Laryngol* [Suppl 11], *83:*27-34, 1974.
13. Bluestone, C.D., Beery, Q.C., and Paradise, J.L.: Audiometry and tympanometry in relation to middle ear effusions in children. *Laryngoscope, 83:*594-604, 1973.
14. Bluestone, C.D., Cantekin, E. I., Beery, Q.C., and Paradise, J.L.: Eustachian tube ventilatory function in relation to cleft palate. *Ann Otol Rhinol Laryngol, 84:*333-339, 1975.
15. Bluestone, C.D., Paradise, J.L., and Beery, Q.C.: Physiology of the Eustachian tube in the pathogenesis and management of middle ear effusions. *Laryngoscope, 82:*1654-1670, 1972.
16. Bluestone, C.D., Paradise, J.L., Beery, Q.C., and Wittel, R.A.: Certain effects of cleft palate repair on Eustachian tube function. *Cleft Palate J, 9:*183-193, 1972.
17. Bluestone, C.D., Wittel, R.A., and Paradise, J.L.: Roentgenographic evaluation of Eustachian tube function in infants with cleft palate and normal palates. *Cleft Palate J, 9:*93-100, 1972.
18. Bluestone, C.D., Wittel, R.A., Paradise, J.L., and Felder, H.: Eustachian tube function as related to adenoidectomy for otitis media. *Trans AAOO, 76:*1325-1339, 1972.
19. Brunck, W.: Die systematische untersuchung des sprachorgans bei angeborenen gaumendefekte. Dissertation, Leipiz, 1906 (from Meissner).
20. Dickson, D.R.: Anatomy of the normal and cleft palate Eustachian tube. *Ann Otol Rhinol Laryngol* [Suppl 25], *85:*24-29, 1976.
21. Donaldson, J.A.: The role of artificial Eustachian tube in cleft palate patients. *Cleft Palate J, 5:*61-66, 1966.
22. Drettner, B.: The nasal airway and hearing in patients with cleft palate. *Acta Otolaryngol, 52:*131-142, 1960.
23. Fara, M. and Dvorak, J.: Abnormal anatomy of the muscles of palatopharyngeal closure in cleft palates. *Plast Reconstr Surg, 46:*488-497, 1970.
24. Flisberg, K., Ingelstedt, S., and Ortegren, U.: Controlled "ear aspiration" of air: A "physiological" test of the tubal function. *Acta Otolaryngol* [Suppl] (Stockh), *82:*35-38, 1963.
25. Flisberg, K., Ingelstedt, S., and Ortegren, U.: I. On middle ear pressure.

Acta Otolaryngol [Suppl], *182*:43-56, 1963.

26. Gaines, E.P.: Frequency and effect of hearing losses in cleft palate cases. *J Speech Hear Disord, 5*:141-149, 1940.
27. Goetzinger, C.P. et al.: Auditory assessment of cleft palate adults. *Acta Otolaryngol* (Stockh), *52*:551-557, 1960.
28. Graham, M.D.: A longitudinal study of ear diseases and hearing loss in patients with cleft lips and palates. *Trans AAOO, 67*:213-222, 1963.
29. Graham, M.D. and Lierle, D.M.: Posterior pharyngeal flap palatoplasty and its relation to ear disease and hearing loss. *Laryngoscope, 72*: 1750-1755, 1962.
30. Gutzman, H.: Zür prognose und Behandlung der angeborenen Gaumendefekte. *Monatsschr Sprachheilkd*, 1893.
31. Halfond, M.M. and Ballenger, J.J.: An audiologic and otorhinologic study of cleft lip and cleft palate cases. *Arch Otolaryngol, 64*:58-62, 1956.
32. Holborow, C.A.: Deafness associated with cleft palate. *J Laryngol Otol, 76*:762-773, 1962.
33. Holborow, C.A.: The assessment of Eustachian tube function. *J Otolaryngol and Soc Aust, 2*:18-20, 1969.
34. Holm, V.A. and Kunze, L.H.: Effect of chronic otitis media on language and speech development. *Pediatrics, 43*:833-839, 1969.
35. Holmes, E.M. and Reed, G.F.: Hearing and deafness in cleft palate patients. *Arch Otolaryngol, 62*:620-624, 1955.
36. Ingelstedt, S. and Ortegren, U.: Qualitative testing of the Eustachian tube function. The snorkel-pressure chamber technique, volumetric determination of tube ventilation. *Acta Otolaryngol* [Suppl], *182*:7-34, 1963.
37. Kriens, O.: Anatomishe untersuchungen am Gespaltenen weich en Gaumen. *Chir Plast Reconstr, 4*:14-32, 1967.
38. Lannois, M.: De l'état de l'oreille moyenne dans les fissures congénitales du palais. *Rev Hebd de Laryngol, 21*:177-184, 1901.
39. Lindsay, W.K., LeMesurier, A.B., and Farmer, A.W.: A study of the speech results of a large series of cleft palate patients. *Plast Reconstr Surg, 27*:273-288, 1962.
40. Linthicum, F.H., Body, H., Keaster, J.: Incidence of middle ear disease in children with cleft palate. *Cleft Palate Bull, 9*:23-25, 1959.
41. Loeb, W.J.: Speech, hearing and the cleft palate. *Arch Otolaryngol, 79*: 20-30, 1964.
42. Lupovich, P., Bluestone, C.D., Paradise, J.L., and Harkins, M.: Middle ear effusions: Preliminary viscometric, histologic and biochemical studies. *Ann Otol Rhinol Laryngol, 80*:342, 1971.
43. Masters, F.W., Bingham, H.G., and Robinson, D.W.: The prevention and treatment of hearing loss in the cleft palate child. *Plast Reconstr Surg, 25*:503-509, 1960.

44. McWilliams, B.J.: Psychological Considerations in the Management of Articulation in Children with Cleft Palate. Presented at the Forty-second Annual Meeting American Speech and Hearing Association, Washington, D.C., November 19-22, 1966.
45. McWilliams, B.J.: Speech and language problems in children with cleft palate. *J Am Med Wom Assoc, 21:*1005, 1966.
46. Means, B.J. and Irwin, J.V.: An analysis of certain measures of intelligence and hearing loss in a sample of Wisconsin cleft palate population. *Cleft Palate Bull, 4:*24, 1954.
47. Meissner, K.: Ohrenerkrankungen bei Gaumenspalten. *Der Hals– Nasen– und Ohrenarzt, 30:*6, 1939.
48. Miller, M.H.: Hearing losses in cleft palate cases: The incidence, type and significance. *Laryngoscope, 66:*1492-1496, 1956.
49. Nassy, E.A.: Hearing Disturbances in Cleft Palate. Dissertation, Amsterdam, 1952.
50. Noone, R.B., Randall, P., Stool, S.E., Hamilton, R., and Winchester, R.A.: The effect on middle ear disease of fracture of the pterygoid hamulus during palatoplasty. *Cleft Palate J, 10:*23-33, 1973.
51. Odoi, H., Proud, G.O., and Toledo, P.S.: Effects of pterygoid hamulotomy upon Eustachian tube function. *Laryngoscope, 81:*1242-1244, 1971.
52. Pannbacker, J.: Hearing loss and cleft palate. *Cleft Palate J, 6:*50-56, 1969.
53. Paparella, M.M., Oda, M., Hiraida, F., and Brady, D.: Pathology of sensorineural hearing loss in otitis media. *Ann Otol Rhinol Laryngol, 81:* 632, 1972.
54. Paradise, J.L. and Bluestone, C.D.: Early treatment of universal otitis media of infants with cleft palate. *Pediatrics, 53:*48-54, 1974.
55. Paradise, J.L., Bluestone, C.D., and Felder, H.: The universality of otitis media in fifty infants with cleft palate. *Pediatrics, 44:*35-42, 1969.
56. Pfisterer, H.: Recent knowledge concerning impairment of hearing in patients with palatal fissure. *HNO, 6:*307, 1958.
57. Ross, M.A.: Functional anatomy of the tensor palati. *Arch Otolaryngol, 93:*1-8, 1971.
58. Sade, J.: Epithelial differentiation. *Ann Otol Rhinol Laryngology,* [Suppl 11], *83:*59-70, 1974.
59. Sataloff, J. and Fraser, M.: Hearing loss in children with cleft palates. *Arch Otolaryngol, 55:*61-64, 1952.
60. Seeler, E.: "Submukose gaumenspalte und Gehor." *Passow-Schafers Beitr, 28:* 1931.
61. Severeid, L.: A longitudinal study of the efficacy of adenoidectomy in children with cleft palate and secretory otitis media. *Trans AAOO, 76:*1319-1324, 1972.
62. Siedentop, K., Tardy, M.E., and Hamilton, L.R.: Eustachian tube function. *Arch Otolaryngol, 88:*386-395, 1968.

63. Skolnik, E.M.: Otologic evaluation in cleft palate patients. *Laryngoscope, 68:*1908-1949, 1958.
64. Smith, R.M. and McWilliams, B.J.: Creative thinking abilities of cleft palate children. *Cleft Palate J, 3:*275, 1966.
65. Soudijn, E.R., Huffstadt, A.J.: Cleft palates and middle ear effusions in babies. *Cleft Palate J, 12:*229-233, 1975.
66. Spriesterbach, D.C. et al.: Hearing loss in children with cleft palates. *Plast Reconstr Surg, 25:*503-509, 1960.
67. Stool, S. and Randall, P.: Unexpected ear disease in infants with cleft palates. *Cleft Palate J, 4:*99-103, 1967.
68. Subtenly, J.D.: Width of nasopharynx and related anatomic structures in normal and unoperated cleft palate children. *Am J Orthod, 41:* 889, 1955.
69. Surina, I. and Jagr, J.: Action potentials of levator and tensor muscles in patients with cleft palate. *Acta Chir Plast, 11:*21-30, 1969.
70. Thomson, H.G. and Harwood-Nash, D.: The fate of the infractured hamuli. *Plast Reconstr Surg, 50:*354-356, 1972.
71. Thorington, J.: Almost total destruction of the velum palati corrected by an artificial soft palate, producing not only greatly improved speech, but an immediate increase of audition. *Med New, 61:*269, 1892; and *Annales du Mal de l'Oreille et du Larynx,* 694, 1892.
72. Variot, G.: Ecoulement de lait par l'oreille d'un nourisson atteint de division congénitale du voile du palais. *Bull Soc de Ped de Paris, 6:* 387, 1904.
73. Walton, W.K.: Audiometrically "normal" conductive hearing losses among the cleft palate. *Cleft Palate J, 10:*99-103, 1973.
74. Whaley, J.B.: Otolaryngologist's role in care of cleft palate patients. *J Can Dent Assoc, 23:*574, 1957.
75. Yules, R.B.: Hearing in cleft palate patients. *Arch Otolaryngol, 91:*319-323, 1970.

—4—

PHARYNGEAL DISEASE AND VELOPHARYNGEAL COMPETENCY AND THEIR RELATIONSHIP TO EAR DISEASE AND HEARING LOSS

LARRY SEVEREID, M.D.

THE PRIMARY CAUSE for the high incidence of ear disease in children with cleft palate is eustachian tube dysfunction.[1,2] The palatal muscles responsible for tubal opening not only have abnormal insertions, but are hypoplastic.[3] Nasopharyngeal disease and velopharyngeal incompetence are two other factors considered to effect tubal function. The unanswered question is not whether they play a role in the production of tubal dysfunction but, rather, to what extent and magnitude. These factors remain points of controversy in the management of cleft palate children, since adenoidectomies for pharyngeal "disease" may result in decreased velopharyngeal closure; early palatal surgery, according to some authors, may result in reduced maxillary growth. In this chapter, the effects of pharyngeal disease and velopharyngeal incompetence upon eustachian tube function will be reviewed.

As in all controversial subjects, one can always find data with conclusions supporting all points of view. The literature relating to cleft palate children and their management is no exception. If one considers the number of medical and surgical variables found in the treatment of these patients and the difficulty controlling these variables when evaluating data, the cause for the controversy is easily understood. Because of the numerous variables, the cause-effect relationship can easily become obscured.

The omission of patient age as a variable may account for many of the contradictory conclusions in the literature. In the evaluation of hearing loss, it has been pointed out that investigators use different definitions of hearing loss, as well as compare patients from different centers where philosophies of medical care differ. Age is one variable that cannot be ignored, if generalizations are to be made about hearing loss in cleft palate children.[4,5] The same consideration should apply to generalizations regarding the different methods of treatment for tubal dysfunction.

PHARYNGEAL DISEASE AND TUBAL DYSFUNCTION

Most of the concepts employed in the management of the cleft palate patient with tubal dysfunction are those used in the noncleft population. A frequent procedure used in children with eustachian tube dysfunction is the adenoidectomy. Those physicians maintaining that adenoid disease contributes to tubal dysfunction believe that the lymphoid tissue either mechanically blocks the tubal orifice or that chronic inflammation produces submucosal edema or hyperplasia of intraluminal lymphoid tissue, resulting in impaired tubal opening.

The primary objection to the removal of the adenoid bed in patients with cleft palates is that velopharyngeal incompetence may be produced or made worse. It has been demonstrated by cinefluoroscopy that the point of palatal contact with the posterior pharyngeal wall is at the level of the adenoid pad.[6] With this fact in mind, a recommended substitution for the adenoidectomy in cleft palate children is the lateral band adenoidectomy.[7,8] This technique should eliminate any lymphoid tissue obstructing the tubal orifice yet maintain the central adenoid pad. The effectiveness of the lateral band adenoidectomy has not been demonstrated.[9] One author opposed to adenoidectomies believes ear disease is more related to impaired nasal airway than to adenoid disease.[10] Other investigators have noted no relationship to adenoid size and ear disease.[11]

Those who favor adenoidectomy in cleft palate children maintain that velopharyngeal closure remains unchanged, and, in many cases, speech is improved.[12,13] With reference to hearing and adenotonsillectomies, one author concluded that the hearing status in the postadenoidectomy group was much improved.[13]

It is apparent that deterioration of speech after adenoidectomy, though not inevitable, is possible. The question remains, "to what extent does the adenoidectomy contribute to establishing normal tubal function?" An attempt to answer this question, based on a retrospective study of cleft palate patients, was undertaken.[14] The records of 160 patients were analyzed. All of these cleft palate patients had at some time shown evidence of eustachian tube dysfunction characterized by reduced hearing acuity or by myringotomy and removal of middle ear effusions. All had, at some time, otologic evidence of immobile, retracted tympanic membranes. The patients had been followed regularly since infancy and up-to-date records were available. The age-range was between five to twenty-seven years (mean, ten years). This longitudinal study permitted one to view the problem of tubal dysfunction and ear disease as a dynamic changing condition, rather than a static one. All but two patients had had transmyrigeal ventilating tubes employed in the management of their hearing loss.

At the time of the study, normal tubal function has been established in 55 percent of the patients: 45 percent still had eustachian tube dysfunction. It must be emphasized that hearing acuity was not used as the indicator of normal tubal function. Instead, evidence of a ventilated middle ear without the presence of a ventilating tube was used. Hearing loss as a result of tympanic membrane changes or ossicular erosion can be present with normal tubal functions and a ventilated middle ear space.

Age of Patient

The importance of age as a variable is appreciated when one separates the patients into age-groups and compares the incidence of tubal dysfunction (Table 4-I). The relationship between patient age and tubal dysfunction is more clearly demonstrated in Figure 4-1. In spite of the fact that all of the patients had, at

TABLE 4-I.
NUMBER AND PERCENT OF SUBJECTS WITH EUSTACHIAN TUBE DYSFUNCTION CLASSIFIED ACCORDING TO AGE

Age in Years	Number of Subjects	Number and Percent With Tubal Dysfunction
5 - 8	88	58 (66%)
9 - 12	24	7 (29%)
13 - 17	34	6 (17%)
18 - 22	10	1 (10%)
23 - 27	4	0 (0%)

From L. Severeid, Longitudinal Study of the Efficacy of Adenoidectomy in Children with Cleft Palate and Secretory Otitis Media, *Transactions of the American Academy of Ophthalmology and Otolaryngology, 76:*1319-1324, 1972. Courtesy of the American Academy of Ophthalmology and Otolaryngology.

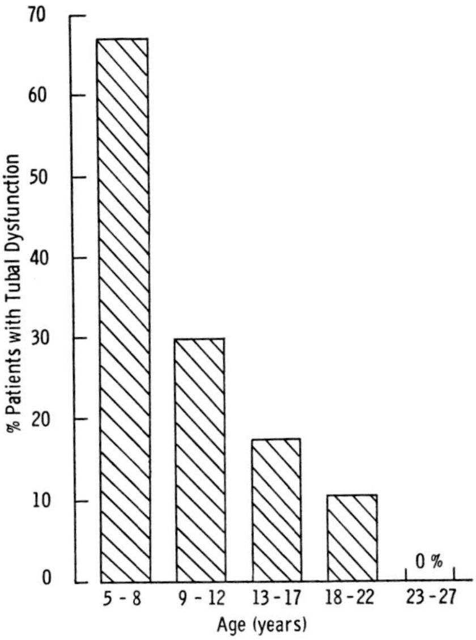

Figure 4-1. Age-group and percent of 160 patients studied who still had tubal dysfunction.

From L. Severeid, Longitudinal Study of the Efficacy of Adenoidectomy in Children with Cleft Palate and Secretory Otitis Media, *Transactions of the American Academy of Opthamology and Otolaryngology, 76:*1319-1324, 1972.

Courtesy of the American Academy of Opthalmology and Otolaryngology.

some time, tubal dysfunction, the number who still exhibited tubal dysfunction decreased as the age increased.

Adenoidectomy

The patients were then divided into two groups: adenoidectomy and nonadenoidectomy. Of the 160 patients, 83 had undergone adenoidectomy. Comparing the two groups, the incidence of tubal dysfunction is higher in the nonadenoidectomy group. This suggests a relationship between the adenoidectomy and the increase in tubal function (Table 4-II). However, examination of Table 4-II reveals that the mean age of the adenoidectomy group is older. When the patients are evaluated by comparison of age-groups, there is no appreciable difference in incidence of tubal dysfunction between the adenoidectomy and nonadenoidectomy patients (Table 4-III). This is more clearly appreciated in Figure 4-2.

If age had been disregarded, one might have assumed that adenoidectomies are responsible for the improved tubal function. In fact, the improved tubal function is more likely related to the increase in age rather than the adenoidectomy.

This study does raise serious question about the efficiency of adenoidectomy as a routine surgical procedure for cleft palate children having tubal dysfunction. It also emphasizes the importance of patient age when analyzing data.

TABLE 4-II.
NUMBER, MEAN AGE, AND PERCENT OF SUBJECTS WITH EUSTACHIAN TUBE DYSFUNCTION CLASSIFIED ACCORDING TO ADENOIDECTOMY.

Group	Number of Subjects	Mean Age (Years)	Number and Percent With Tubal Dysfunction
Adenoidectomy	83	11	32 (38%)
Non-adenoidectomy	77	9	40 (52%)

From L. Severeid, Longitudinal Study of the Efficacy of Adenoidectomy in Children with Cleft Palate and Secretory Otitis Media, *Transactions of the American Academy of Ophthalmology and Otolaryngology, 76:*1319-1324, 1972. Courtesy of the American Academy of Ophthalmology and Otolaryngology.

TABLE 4-III.
NUMBER AND PERCENT OF SUBJECTS IN THE TWO GROUPS (ADENOIDECTOMY AND NON-ADENOIDECTOMY) WITH EUSTACHIAN TUBE DYSFUNCTION LISTED ACCORDING TO AGE.

	Adenoidectomy		Non-adenoidectomy	
Age in Years	Number of Patients	Number and Percent With Tubal Dysfunction	Number of Patients	Number and Percent With Tubal Dysfunction
5-8	31	21 (67%)	57	37 (66%)
9-12	18	5 (28%)	6	2 (33%)
13-17	25	5 (20%)	9	1 (11%)
18-22	7	1 (14%)	3	0 (0%)
23-27	2	0 (0%)	2	0 (0%)

From L. Severeid, Longitudinal Study of the Efficacy of Adenoidectomy in Children with Cleft Palate and Secretory Otitis Media, *Transactions of the American Academy of Ophthalmology and Otolaryngology, 76:*1319-1324, 1972. Courtesy of the American Academy of Ophthalmology and Otolaryngology.

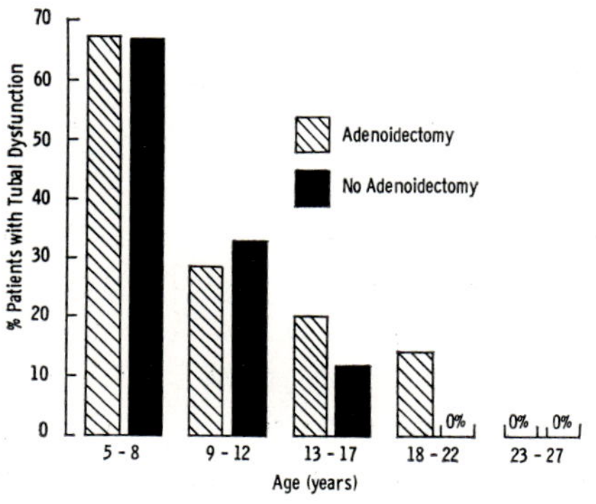

Figure 4-2. Percent of subjects (adenoidectomy and non-adenoidectomy) with eustachian tube dysfunction listed according to age.

From L. Severeid, Longitudinal Study of the Efficacy of Odenoidectomy in Children with Cleft Palate and Secretory Otitis Media, *Transactions of the American Academy of Ophthalmology and Otolaryngology, 76:*1319-1324, 1972.

Courtesy of the American Academy of Opthalmology and Otolaryngology.

Adenoidectomy, as a treatment for tubal dysfunction in cleft palate patients, probably should be reserved for selected cases where there is obvious encroachment upon the tubal orifice.

VELOPHARYNGEAL INCOMPETENCE AND EUSTACHIAN TUBE DYSFUNCTION

The relationship between velopharyngeal incompetence and eustachian tube dysfunction appears to be more positive. Restoration of the velopharyngeal sphincteric mechanism has been clearly correlated to improved hearing acuity.[2,12,15] Because of the observation, many authors have advocated early closure of the palatal cleft.[9,16] The primary objection to early closure of the hard palatal defect is the implication that there is impairment of bony growth resulting in a more significant facial deformity.[17,18] Other investigators do not agree with this opinion and contend that there is no difference in maxillary growth between those patients who have had early palatoplasties and those who have had delayed procedures.[19,20]

Reflux of oral contents into the nasopharynx occurs in the child with an unrepaired palate and may result in inflammation and edema around the tubal orifice. In addition, the abnormal muscle insertions of the unrepaired cleft palate are considered to be unfavorable for normal tubal opening. Reestablishment of the normal sphincteric mechanism of the velopharynx not only results in protection of the tubal orifices from the oral cavity but may establish a more normal muscular mechanism for tubal opening. Simply closing the cleft may be helpful in establishing better tubal function, but some surgeons report that an elongation procedure combined with the palatal closure not only results in improved velopharyngeal competence but improved hearing.[9] Retrodisplacement of the levator muscles in previously repaired but incompetent palates has also resulted in improved velopharyngeal closure and, in some instances, improved eustachian tube function.[21] It remains unclear whether the reported improved tubal function occurs as a result of improved velopharyngeal closure or because of the improved tubal muscle dynamics.

Palatal Obturators and Hearing Loss

Numerous studies have indicated that the incidence of hearing loss is greater in patients who wear palatal obturators.[2,9,12,22] Since the obturator effectively separates the nasopharynx from the oropharynx, this would suggest that the cause for the increased incidence of the hearing loss is from the impaired palatal muscle dynamics.

There is no evidence that the obturator encroaches upon the tubal orifices or prevents them from opening.[23] In this study of a series of patients whose clefts had been managed by palatal obturation, it was noted that the postobturator hearing status remained the same or improved. In this study, no attempt was made to compare the hearing status of obturated patients with a comparable group of patients who had palatoplasties, but it was pointed out that no deterioration in hearing occurred when palatal obturation was employed.

Pharyngeal Flaps and Hearing Loss

The primary surgical procedure employed in the management of velopharyngeal incompetence following palatoplasty is the posterior pharyngeal flap. Theoretically, the superiorly based flap might be assumed to interfere with normal tubal function. Studies comparing presurgical with the postsurgical hearing indicate that the hearing levels are no worse and are frequently better.[19,24] This would indicate that there is a positive relationship between improved eustachian tube function and velopharyngeal competence.

Eustachian Tube Function and Hearing Acuity

Most studies dealing with ear disease in cleft palate children have used hearing acuity as the indicator of the problem. This is appropriate, considering that hearing, after all, is the primary concern. Hearing acuity, however, is not a perfect indicator of normal tubal function. The hearing may be normal in patients who have nonfunctioning eustachian tubes, if indwelling transmyringeal ventilating tubes are used or small perforations are present.

Of equal importance, a patient may have established normal eustachian tube function, but, because of previous tubal dysfunction, irreversible changes may have occurred to the tympanic membrane or ossicular chain, producing a hearing loss.

The goal of the otolaryngologist should be to protect the sound-conducting mechanism in the cleft palate patient by preventing the irreversible changes that may occur to the middle ear in the presence of a nonfunctioning eustachian tube. Maintaining a ventilated middle ear by using the transmyringeal ventilating tube remains the mainstay in the management of tubal dysfunction until the normal function is established.

It is important to remember that time is an important variable, when evaluating any surgical variable (adenoidectomy, palatoplasty, pharyngeal flap) and its relationship to improved eustachian tube function. Improved hearing and improved tubal function is related to the progression of age.[5,14,25] One cannot conclude that improved hearing has resulted from any surgical procedure, unless the results are compared with a control group of patients of similar age. The dilemma faced in assessing the cause-effect relationship in the management of patients with tubal dysfunction can best be characterized in the quotation by John Kentish from his essay on burns given in 1797.

> It falls to the lot of few men to appreciate properly the effect of various modes of treatment in a particular disease; for if the patient recovers, whatever was the treatment, whether good or bad, we flatter ourselves it was the effect of our superior merit in conducting the disease; but future experience may convince us the recovery, of which we so vainly boosted, was a victory of nature over the malpractice of art.

REFERENCES

1. Bluestone, C.D., Wittel, R.A., and Paradise, J.L.: Roentgenographic evaluation of eustachian tube function in infants with cleft and normal palates. *Cleft Palate J,* 9:93-100, Ap. 1972.
2. Paulsen, J.W.: Studies on the hearing and tubal function in a series of children with cleft palates. *Acta Otolaryngol* [Suppl], (Stockh)., *188,* 1964.
3. Fara, M. and Dvorak, J.: Abnormal anatomy of the muscles of palatopharyngeal closure in cleft palates. *Plast Reconstr Surg, 48:*488-497, Nov. 1970.

4. Spriestersbach, D.C., Lierle, D.M., Moll, K.L., and Prather, W.F.: Hearing loss in children with cleft palates. *Plast Reconstr Surg, 30:*336-347, Sept. 1962 .
5. Graham, M.D.: A longitudinal study of ear disease and hearing loss in patients with cleft lips and palates. *Ann Otol, 73:*34-46, March 1964.
6. Calnan, J.S.: Modern views of passavant's ridge. *Br J Plast Surg, 10:*89-113, July 1957.
7. Subtelney, J.D. and Baker, H.K.: The significance of adenoid tissue in velopharyngeal function. *Plast Reconstr Surg, 17:*235-257, 1956.
8. Berner, R.E.: Hazards of adenotonsillectomy in the child with cleft palate. *JAMA, 181:*558-559, Aug. 1962.
9. Masters, F.W., Bingham, H.G., and Robinson, D.S.: The prevention and treatment of hearing loss in the cleft palate child. *Plast Reconstr Surg, 25:*502-509, May 1960.
10. Drettner, B.: The nasal airway and hearing in patients with cleft palate. *Acta Otolaryngol, 52:*131, 1961.
11. Holmes, E.M. and Reed, G.F.: Hearing and deafness in cleft palate patients. *Arch Otolaryngol, 62:*620-624, Dec. 1955.
12. Loeb, W.J.: Speech, hearing and the cleft palate. *Arch Otolaryngol, 79:* 4-14, 1964.
13. Chalat, N.I.: Tonsillectomy, adenoidectomy and the cleft palate clinic. *Laryngoscope, 75:*408-427, March 1971.
14. Severeid L.: Longitudinal study of the efficacy of adenoidectomy in children with cleft palate and secretory otitis media. *Tr Am Acad Opthalmol Otolaryngol, 76:*1319-1324, Sept.-Oct. 1972.
15. Yules, R.B.: Hearing in cleft palate patients. *Arch Otolaryngol, 91:*319-323, Ap 1970.
16. Glover, D.M.: A long range valuation of cleft palate repair. *Plast Reconstr Surg, 27:*19-30, 1961.
17. Dingman, R.O. and Grabb, W.C.: A rational program for surgical management of bil. cleft lip and palate. *Plast Reconstr Surg, 47:*239-242, March 1971.
18. Bernstein, L.: The effect of timing of cleft palate operations on subsequent growth of maxilla, *78:*1510-1565, Sept. 1968.
19. Mazaheri, M., Harding, R.L., and Nanda, S.: The Effect of Surgery on Maxillary Growth and Cleft Width. *Plast Reconstr Surg, 40:*22-30, Jul. 1969.
20. Alexander, H.B., Moore, A.W., and Coe, H.E.: The Time and Chance for Repair of Cleft Palate in Relation to the Type of Surgical Repair and its Effect on Bony Growths of the Face. *Plast Reconstr Surg, 18:* 469-473, Dec. 1956.
21. Edgerton, M.T. and Sellion, A. Lee: Surgical retrodisplacement of the levator veli palatine muscle. *Plast Reconstr Surg, 47:*154-167.
22. Skolnik, M.S.: Otologic evaluation of cleft palate patients. *Laryngoscope, 68:*1908-1949, Nov. 1958.

23. Graham, M.D., Schweiger, J.W., and Oein, W.D.: Hearing loss and ear disease in cleft palate patients with obturators. *Plast Reconstr Surg, 30:*348-358, Sept. 1962.

24. Graham, M.D. and Lierle, D.M.: Posterior pharyngeal flap palatoplasty and its relationship to ear disease and hearing loss. *Laryngoscope, 72:* 1750-1755, Dec. 1962.

25. Goetzinger, C.P., Embrey, J.E., Brooks, R.B., and Proud, G.O.: Auditory assessment of cleft palate adults. *Acta Otolaryngol* (Stockh), *52:*551, 1961.

—5—

HISTOPATHOLOGY OF THE MIDDLE EAR

Fred H. Linthicum Jr., M.D.

The histologic picture in the middle ear of patients with cleft palates can vary from normal to total destruction of the middle ear cleft either by cholesteatoma (Plate 1-1) or complete fibrosis (Plate 1-2). The latter two situations should be preventable with adequate medical and surgical therapy.

Middle Ear Effusion

This is the most common abnormal finding in the middle ear of patients with cleft palates. This fluid is usually a transudate rather than an exudate and is the result of an extravasation of fluid from the mucosa and blood vessels of the middle ear into the middle ear. This is due to the persistent negative pressure resulting from the failure of the eustachian tube to open and ventilate the ear. The air in the middle ear is continuously being absorbed according to the physical law of gases exposed to a liquid (mucus), i.e. they dissolve into the liquid according to their partial pressure. This negative pressure not only produces an extravasation into the middle ear but also edema of the middle ear mucosa and tubotympanum.

The effusion when it first occurs is usually serous. The mucosa is somewhat edematous (Plate 1-3). If the effusion persists for months or years, it gradually thickens, and the mucosa actually hypertrophies. Occasionally, the mucosa will undergo a metaplastic change to a secretory ciliated columnar epithelium (Plate 1-4). This produces the true secretory otitis media: the ear that continues to exude sterile mucus through a ventilation tube when such is placed in the tympanic membrane. The entire middle ear and mastoid may undergo this metaplasia. This condition, true secretory otitis media, is also known as *serous mastoiditis.*

The picture of long-standing middle ear effusion, i.e. thickened fluid and hypertrophied mucosa, may also occur as the result of treatment of an acute otitis media with antibiotics. The medication sterilizes the pus in the middle ear, which persists as a glue-like material. The inflammatory response of the mucosa is, again, hypertrophy, and occasionally, metaplasia.

Persistent middle ear effusion predisposes to recurrent otitis media, due to the fact that the effusion is an excellent culture medium. These repeated attacks of otitis media may well produce progressive damage to the tympanic membrane and ossicular chain.

Cholesterol Granuloma

On occasion, bleeding will occur into the middle ear fluid. After several weeks, the erythrocytes degenerate, liberating cholesterol into the fluid. The cholesterol becomes a foreign body and stimulates a typical foreign body reaction consisting of granulation tissue, round cells, and multinucleated giant cells (Plate 1-5.) The granulation tissue increases and surrounds the middle ear effusion, separating it into numerous small cysts containing cholesterol crystals appearing as golden flakes (Plate 1-6). These same golden flakes will be found in the granulation tissue itself (Plate 2-1). Concurrently, there is the same metaplasia of the usually low-cuboidal epithelium of posterior middle ear cleft and mastoid into a secretory ciliated columnar epithelium (Plate 2-2). Gradually, the granulation tissue will undergo fibrosis. This will eventually lead to a complete replacement of the middle ear cleft and mastoid air spaces by fibrous tissue, a condition which, so far, has been uncorrectable surgically or medically.

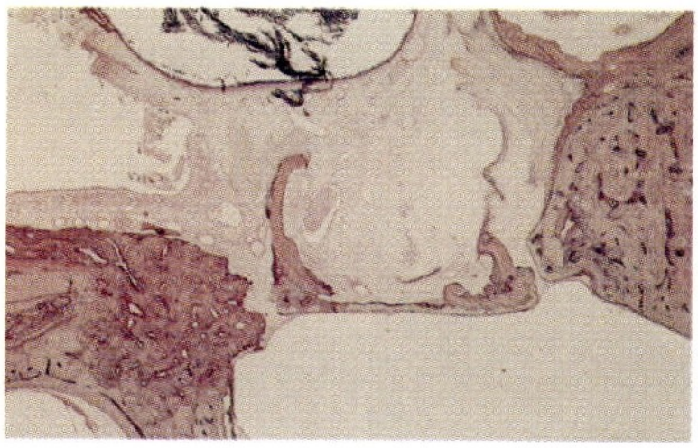

Plate 1-1.

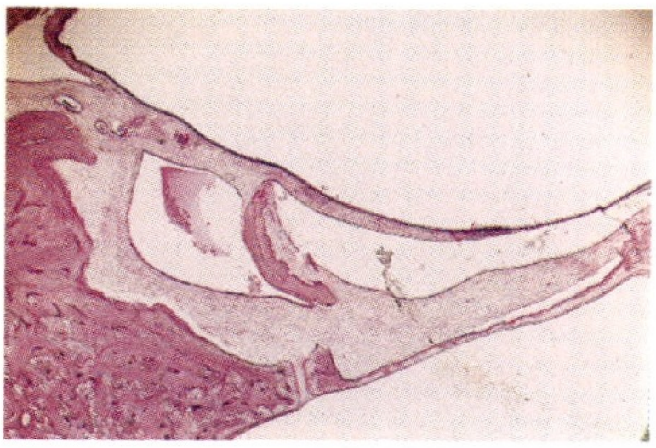

Plate 1-2.

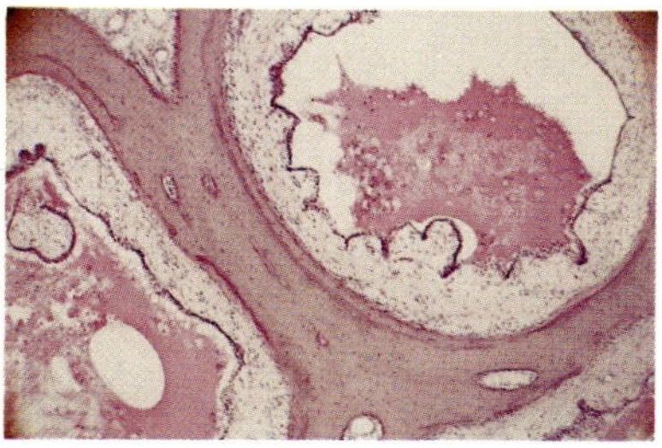

Plate 1-3.

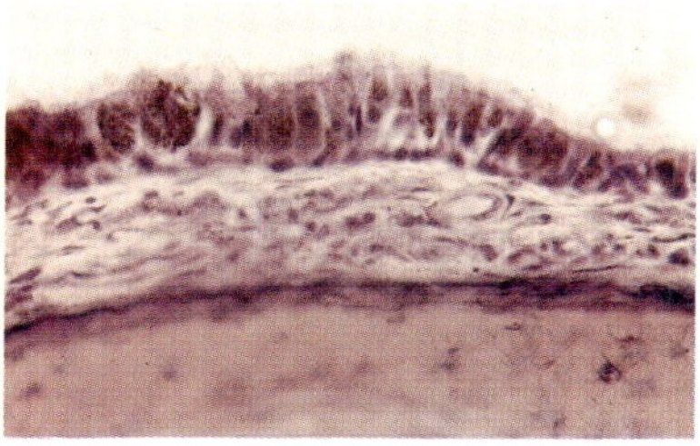

Plate 1-4.

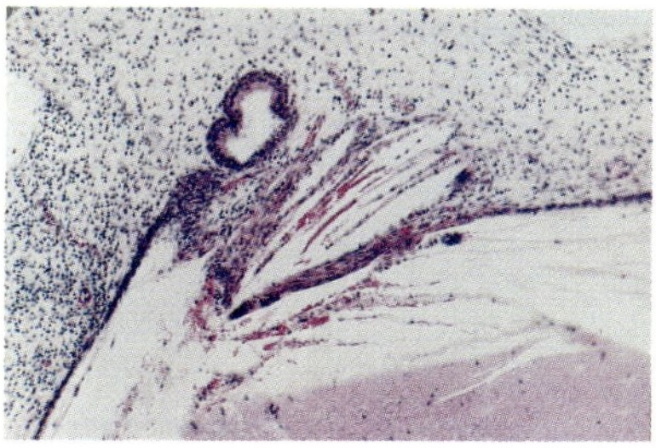

Plate 1-5.

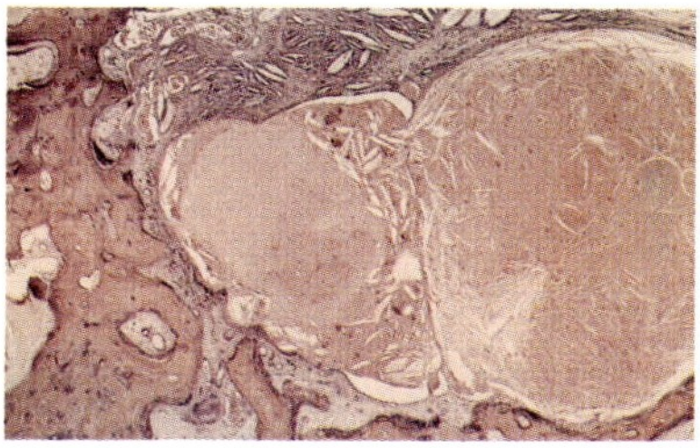

Plate 1-6.

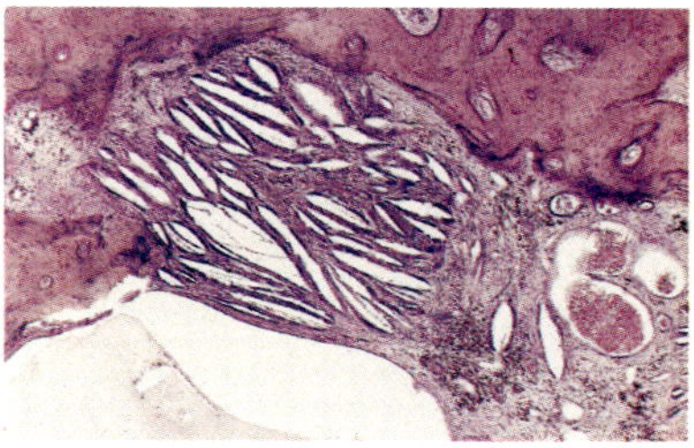

Plate 2-1.

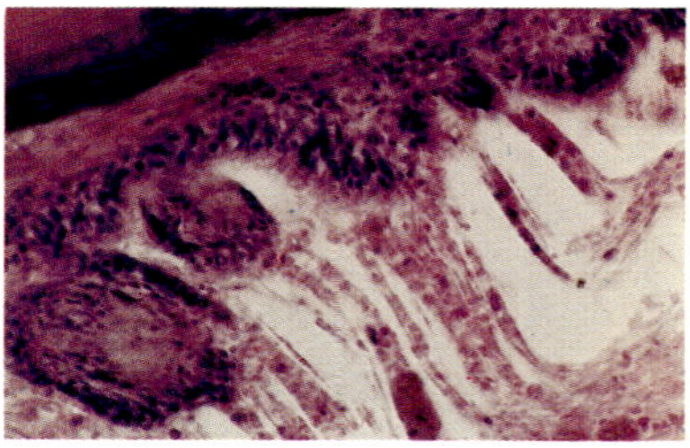

Plate 2-2.

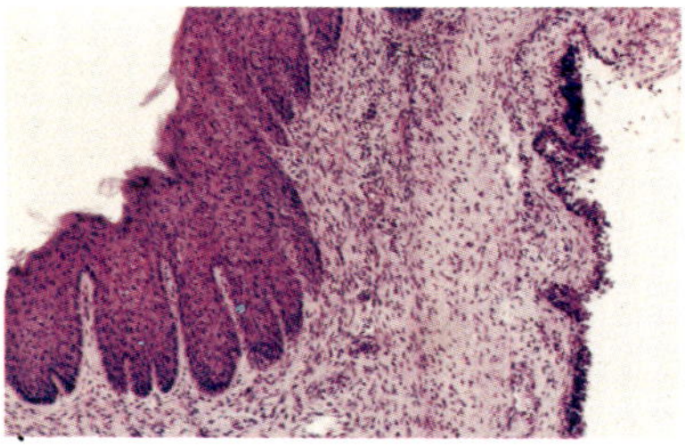

Plate 2-3.

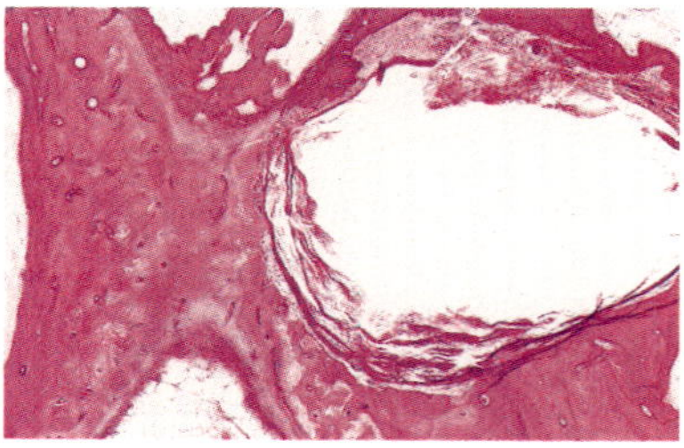

Plate 2-4.

Primary Acquired Cholesteatoma

The eustachian tube is often inadequate in cleft palate patients in ventilating the middle ear early in life. This delays absorption of mesenchyme in the middle ear, especially in the epitympanum. The presence of this persistent mesenchyme allows the rete pegs of the squamous epithelium of the pars flaccida to penetrate it, as there is no fibrous layer in this portion of the tympanic membrane (Plate 2-3). One or more of these pegs may become isolated from the squamous epithelium on the surface of the pars flaccida (Plate 2-4). This gradually enlarges to fill the ear cleft below the level of the chorda tympani, destroying bone and ossicles as it does so. It may become manifest only after an acute otitis media causes infection of the cholesteatoma and its rupture through the tympanic membrane. On the other hand, the only evidence of the existence of such a condition may be a conductive hearing loss and a pale area behind an intact tympanic membrane that otherwise has the appearance of a simple middle ear effusion.

Secondary Acquired Cholesteatoma

Repeated perforations resulting from acute otitis media or insertion of ventilation tubes frequently result in a thin, atrophic scar in the tympanic membrane. The persistent negative pressure causing the recurrent otitis media or persistent middle ear effusion also tends to produce a retraction of this atrophic membrane. The sac produced is lined with desquamating squamous epithelium, which tends to accumulate. If not carefully evacuated or corrected surgically, such a sac is gradually retracted into the middle ear, epitympanum, and antrum, thus producing a secondary acquired cholesteatoma.

Congenital Ossicular Deformities

The anomaly of cleft palate may also be accompanied by congenital abnormalities of the middle ear cleft. These may include anomalies of the malleus, such as fixation, distortion of the incus, a lack of an incostapedial articulation, absence of the stapedial cura, or fixation of the stapedial footplate. Not infrequently, the stapedius tendon is lacking. In these cases, the facial nerve may be in an aberrant course.

Some cases of cleft palate are also accompanied by a complete aplasia of the external auditory canal. Most often, these patients have a sufficient middle ear cleft and mastoid air system. The malleus is usually fixed to the lateral wall of the epitympanum. The other ossicles may be likewise deformed. The facial nerve usually is in an abnormal position.

The tympanic bone or the external auditory canal and the tympanic bone may be represented as a solid plug of bone or may be absent, and the temporomandibular joint may occupy the normal space of the tympanic bone. Occasionally, a concommitant middle ear effusion may exist due to the malfunctioning eustachian tube.

The histopathologic changes in the middle ear of patients with submucous cleft are no different than those in other patients with poorly functioning eustachian tubes, but occur much more frequently.

—6—

OTOLOGIC ASSESSMENT AND MANAGEMENT OF THE CLEFT PALATE INDIVIDUAL

MALCOLM D. GRAHAM, M.D.

WHILE EAR DISEASE and hearing losses have been recognized as frequent complications associated with the congenital cleft palate deformity, it remained for Paradise and Bluestone[1] in 1969 to show this association to be almost without exception. Thus, it is incumbent on physicians, audiologists, speech therapists, dentists, social workers, and educators to be aware of this relationship and be alert to its occurrence, treatment, recurrence, and long-term management.

The birth of an infant with a congenital cleft palate should alert the physician to the necessity for an otologic assessment to determine whether or not otitis media is present. Frequent re-examination at regular intervals, e.g. every three months, will then allow prompt institution of therapy when disease becomes manifest and permit prompt recognition of recurrent problems should they occur. While it is not possible to assess the hearing of the newborn accurately, the experienced audiologist will soon be able to determine free-field hearing levels and by early childhood have accurate threshold levels for each ear. The objective audiometric techniques currently being developed may soon permit early and accurate thresholds of hearing for each ear.

This chapter will detail the otologic assessment and management of the individual with the cleft palate deformity.

GENERAL MEDICAL HISTORY

The infant born with a cleft palate, with or without a cleft lip, will universally be subject to ear disease. However, if the cleft lip deficit alone exists, the prevalence of ear disease is the same as in the child not so afflicted.[2] Thus, making this differentiation is of clinical importance. The age of the individual when first seen is also important. If an infant, otitis media will invariably occur; if the individual is an adult, the likelihood of further or continuing problems from ear disease is small indeed.

The presence of additional abnormalities is of importance. Cardiovascular or neurological deficits may be life-threatening and, therefore, take precedence in treatment over ear disease. The child's intelligence will determine his learning capabilities and will predicate his ability to proceed satisfactorily in school, particularly if a hearing loss is present. The extent of the cleft lip and/or palate will determine the extent and frequency of surgical procedures which the child must undergo. These interventions may influence the routine follow-up examinations of the ears and may require greater flexibility in scheduling and much persistence in assuring that otologic care continues.

OTOLOGIC HISTORY

The individual's otologic history may be of great importance. Has there been acute or chronic ear disease? Has the individual had pain, drainage from the ear, hearing loss, or surgery upon the ear?

If the child has not had previous otologic assessment and care, there may well be otitis media or the stigmata or chronic ear disease, with or without attendant hearing loss. Treatment may be made difficult by adhesive or chronic inflammatory ear disease.

If the individual has received prior otologic care, the nature of this care is of importance. Have myringotomies been performed? Have polyethylene tubes been inserted? If so, how often and was there ear drainage thereafter? Has reconstructive or mastoid surgery been performed? Finally, have the tonsils and adenoids been removed? If not, have these been infected? The presence and the consequence of possible future removal of the tonsils and adenoids must be taken into consideration in the planning for future palatal surgery and later speech therapy.

GENERAL OTOLARYNGOLOGIC EXAMINATION

The presence of the cleft palate and its degree of severity should be recorded on standard diagram forms available for this purpose. If surgery has been performed, a record should be made of the type of surgery and the age at which it was performed. An idea can thus be gained of the results of past treatment and the need for future surgery.

The size of the tonsils and adenoids should be recorded and the degree of nasal reflux noted. If the reflux is great, there is often nasal mucosal hyperemia and edema. The size of the nasal turbinates is of importance in that these structures may be providing adequate speech quality in the face of significant velopharyngeal incompetency.

OTOLOGIC EXAMINATION

In order to adequately examine the ear, optimal conditions for examination must be available. The examination room should be equipped with an otoscope, various-sized ear speculi, instruments for the removal of wax and debris from the ear canal, suction apparatus, pneumatic otoscope, and a surgical microscope.

Initially, the ear should be inspected without magnification to detect scars and evidence of congenital deformities. The pneumatic otoscope should then be used, and finally, the surgical microscope. The pneumatic otoscope should be employed regularly to determine tympanic membrane and malleolar mobility.

Tympanic Membrane

The tympanic membrane's appearance is of paramount importance. From its appearance, the experienced clinician can tell much concerning the past history of ear disease and the present activity of the disease process and can often gain a general impression as to the level of hearing. Additionally, the eustachian tube function can be deduced and an idea formulated of the treatment required for the elimination of ear disease and hearing loss, should these be present.

Various tympanic membrane appearances may be encountered, and many are illustrated in this book.

Perforation

The perforation may be central or marginal. The central perforation has a margin of tympanic membrane around it and usually is not associated with cholesteatoma. The ear, if draining, will usually respond to local treatment. Marginal perforations usually are located peripherally in the posterior one half of the tympanic membrane and often are associated with cholesteatoma. These ears frequently have a malodorous discharge and may not respond to local treatment.

Retraction

Here the tympanic membrane is intact, but it is displaced medially toward the middle ear. The tympanic membrane may be mobile or fixed to the underlying ossicles or medial wall of the middle ear. The pneumatic otoscope is particularly helpful in making this differentiation, especially if used in conjunction with the operating microscope. Neither the presence nor degree of retraction can be correlated with the degree of hearing loss, for it is not unusual to see marked degrees of retraction with normal or near-normal hearing. Retraction is frequently encountered in the presence of fluid in the middle ear, and is the most commonly seen abnormality of the tympanic membrane in the cleft palate individual. Retraction usually results from eustachian tube insufficiency which, if prolonged in duration, may lead to atrophy of the tympanic membrane and eventually to a condition known as *atelectasis of the tympanic membrane.*

Atelectasis of the Tympanic Membrane

The tympanic membrane is said to be atelectatic when it is both thinned and markedly retracted. It usually results from prolonged eustachian tube insufficiency and should seldom be seen in the cleft palate individual, if the ears have been adequately treated and reexamined at regular intervals.

Inflammation

The normal tympanic membrane is not only mobile but also translucent. This allows the examiner to detect fluid or a mass in the middle ear. However, in acute otitis media, the tympanic membrane may be thickened and very inflamed. In the earlier stages of acute otitis media, only the tympanic membrane is involved, but with further progression of the inflammatory process, pus accumulates in the middle ear behind the tympanic membrane. Eventually, if untreated, the tympanic membrane may rupture, allowing the pus to escape into the external auditory canal.

Tympanosclerosis and Scarring

These conditions may exist separately or simultaneously, both with or without a tympanic membrane perforation. *Tympanosclerosis* is a hyaline degeneration of the connective tissue in the tympanic membrane and is frequently seen after prolonged inflammation of the ear. However, it may be seen without the individual having been aware of ear disease. Thickening and scarring of the tympanic membrane is frequently seen, and while there is seldom impairment of the motion of the tympanic membrane, it may become markedly less translucent, thereby precluding an accurate assessment of the middle ear condition.

While the appearance of the tympanic membrane tells much about the condition of the ear and the degree of hearing loss, the temptation to relate appearance of the tympanic membrane to hearing level must be resisted, particularly in the older child or adult, for it has been shown that great variation exists in these relationships.[2]

Discharge

The presence of a purulent discharge from the ear canal is an indication of an ear infection. The discharge may be profuse or scanty or there may be merely a purulent crusting in the deep ear canal. If crusts are present, they must be removed to allow inspection for underlying infection, granulations, or cholesteatoma. A mucoid discharge is usually an indication of eustachian tube dysfunction, allergy, or mucosal disease. This discharge may be thin or thick and tenacious.

Cholesteatoma

Cholesteatoma may be described as the accumulation of exfoliated keratin in the middle ear or other pneumatized areas of the temporal bone arising from keratinized squamous epithelium that has invaded these areas from the external auditory canal.[3] Numerous theories of origin are held; these are completely summarized by Shambaugh.[4]

In the cleft palate individual, it is unusual to encounter cholesteatoma, even in the presence of chronic ear infection and perforation. However, it appears that eustachian tube insufficiency so commonly found in the cleft palate child may be a significant contributing factor in the development of cholesteatoma. While this may be insidious and asymptomatic, eventually a purulent, malodorous discharge from the ear canal occurs. Local therapy may eliminate this infection, but frequently, in the advanced stages, only surgical intervention for the removal of the cholesteatoma will result in the elimination of this disease process.

Thus, it is clear that accurate assessment of the tympanic membrane is of paramount importance in the ear examination and the findings should be recorded in detail in a universally understandable way. Recently, the Committee on Epidemiology of the National Otitis Media Conference, under the Chairmanship of Ralph E. Naunton, M.D., drew up guidelines for recording these findings.[5] The recommended recording method is detailed in Figure 6-1.

Middle Ear Status

When viewed through a perforation, the middle ear mucosa and ossicular chain are often visible. Particularly when utilizing the magnification provided by the surgical microscope, the mucosal appearance is clearly seen, and the presence or absence

SCHEMA FOR DESCRIBING OTOSCOPIC FINDINGS

1. Perforations
   - Presence or absence
   - Site
     - Pars tensa
       - Marginal
       - Central
     - Pars flaccida (include retraction)
   - Size
   - Moist or dry
   - Cholesteatoma seen or not

2. Mobility

	Tympanic Membrane	*Ossicles*
Mobile		
Partly mobile		
Immobile		

3. Scarring

		Fibrosis	*Atrophy**	*Tympano-sclerosis*
Small	up to 1/3			
Medium	up to 2/3			
Large	up to 3/3			

*Term includes healed perforation and monomeric membrane

4. Plane of pars tensa
   - Bulging
   - Normal
   - Retracted
     - Moderate (retracted without touching medial wall)
     - Severe (touching medial wall)

5. Color
   - Normal (for age and race)
   - Abnormal (exclude injection and tympanosclerotic plaques)

Figure 6-1.

of mucoid discharge ascertained. The long process of the malleus and incus, as well as the entire stapes, may be inspected and their mobility determined by palpation. Tympanosclerosis involving the middle ear mucosa and/or the ossicles can be seen. Often the presence and extent of granulation tissue and cholesteatoma involvement of the middle ear and epitympanum can be determined.

The status of the middle ear, when visualized through the perforation, is important, not only to allow the otologist to design a course of treatment, but also to allow a more accurate prognostication of the outcome of future surgery to eliminate ear disease and reverse hearing loss.

While accurate hearing assessment is not usually possible in infancy, once the child is two to three years old, fairly reliable free-field assessment can be obtained. This allows a prediction of whether or not the learning process will be seriously affected. By the time the child is of kindergarten age, an accurate threshold for each ear has usually been established.

Usually the hearing loss, if present, is conductive in type and, therefore, potentially reversible. Because it is usually bilateral, it places a greater urgency on the need for early recognition and treatment in order to prevent the learning problems associated with the hearing loss in these individuals.

Careful pure tone and speech tests should be performed routinely and the test results confirmed by employing the standard tuning fork tests. In this manner, the type of hearing loss present, conductive, sensorineural, or mixed, can be ascertained. The results to be expected by medical or surgical management can be predicted, and anticipated learning problems can be predicated.

RADIOGRAPHIC EVALUATION

While the infant or young child will not have radiographic assessment prior to myringotomy and ventilation tube insertion, nevertheless, in the older child or adult, mastoid x rays are often of value. The degree of mastoid pneumatization and the presence or absence of attic erosion can be ascertained by the routine Stenvers, Laws, and base view tests. If a more detailed assessment of the middle ear, cochlea, vestibular system, internal auditory canals, or petrous apex are desired, anteroposterior and lateral polytomes of the petrous pyramid are useful. While the treatment plan is seldom based on x-ray findings, nevertheless occasional unsuspected, associated diseases are present, and the otolaryngologist should be aware of this abnormality early in the course of management. The most frequent abnormality reported on radiographic examination of the cleft palate individual is cloudiness of the mastoid air cells. This may lead to the suspicion that an acute mastoiditis is present. However, this radiographic appearance is usually created by fluid in the middle ear and mastoid air cell system and not by the cell breakdown, as seen in acute mastoiditis.

OTOLOGIC DISEASES

While otologic disease in cleft palate individuals is universal, the residual serious otologic consequences of acute and chronic inflammatory disease and the resultant hearing loss are largely preventable. Therefore, a thorough understanding and appreciation of the ear diseases and resultant hearing loss found in the cleft palate individual would appear to be valuable to all therapists involved in the treatment of the individual with a cleft palate.

Otitis media is an inflammation of the middle ear space and its extensions. There follows the classification recommended by the 1970 National Otitis Media Conference.[5]

A. Nonsuppurative (serous, mucous, or hemorrhagic)
   1. Acute
   2. Chronic
B. Suppurative (with or without perforation)
   1. Acute
   2. Chronic
      a. Active
      b. Inactive

The cleft palate individual may suffer from any or all forms of otitis media at various times.

Nonsuppurative Otitis Media

This condition results in the accumulation of sterile fluid in the middle ear space with or without the history of ear infection.

Nonsuppurative otitis media is the most frequent form of ear disease found in the individual with a cleft palate. The fluid may be thin and amber colored or thick and grey colored. A more uncommon variant is hemorrhagic; the fluid may be thin or thick. Children with nonsuppurative otitis media frequently are asymptomatic. They usually have a significant conductive hearing loss secondary to the dampening effect of the fluid on the tympanic membrane and ossicles. Ear pain may accompany this fluid accumulation, if the process began as an inflammatory one. In the older child or adult, fullness, a plugged sensation in the ear, decreased hearing, and slight dizziness or tinnitus may be noticed. Upon examination, the appearance of the tympanic membrane varies greatly.

If the middle ear is only partially filled with thin serous fluid, an air fluid level will be visible, often with bubbles evident in the fluid. However, usually the middle ear is completely filled with fluid, and these previous findings are not evident. The tympanic membrane appears amber colored and loses its translucency. If the fluid is mucoid, the tympanic membrane appears more grayish and, if hemorrhagic, the fluid is bluish or dull gray. The blood vessels of the tympanic membrane along the handle of the malleus and circumferentially around the tympanic membrane are often dilated and, most characteristic of the middle ear, filled with mucoid fluid. Mobility of the tympanic membrane is impaired, a feature readily noticeable when the pneumatic otoscope is used while the tympanic membrane is observed under the surgical microscope. Characteristic of the presence of mucoid fluid in the middle ear is a wrinkling appearance of the tympanic membrane while attempting to move it with the pneumatic otoscope. Because the tympanic membrane is intact, there is no drainage. Additionally, pain is usually absent, thereby leading the inexperienced examiner to consider the tympanic membrane normal, while a very significant bilateral conductive hearing loss may be present.

Suppurative Otitis Media

The acute form of suppurative otitis media often accompanies an upper respiratory infection and usually is characterized by pain and temperature elevation. Should the tympanic membrane rupture, discharge from the ear canal follows. The acute infection usually responds rapidly to antibiotic therapy. However, a myringotomy may be required if pain is severe and bulging of the tympanic membrane is present. This procedure will give dramatic and prompt relief of pain. However, the acute infection may leave the middle ear filled with fluid and, thus, a chronic condition ensues. Should a tympanic membrane perforation not heal, or should retraction of the tympanic membrane or cholesteatoma formation occur, then the suppurative otitis media is considered chronic. These are fairly frequent features of ear disease in the cleft palate individual. If active purulent discharge from the ear occurs, or if cholesteatoma debris accumulates, then chronic otitis media is considered active. If, on the other hand, the ear is dry, notwithstanding the underlying pathology, it is referred to as being inactive.

The prime symptom of acute otitis media is pain. However, in infancy, this pattern may vary. Crying of the infant, fever of unknown origin, lethargy, or unexplained diarrhea may alert the examiner to the presence of acute otitis media.

The appearance of the tympanic membrane in acute suppurative otitis media varies greatly. Initially, there is a lack of luster and a slight thickening of the tympanic membrane. Dilation of the blood vessels on the tympanic membrane then occurs, and hyperemia follows. Later, a pus accumulation in the middle ear results in a bulging of the tympanic membrane and the loss of all normal landmarks. These stages may evolve with extreme rapidity and only a few hours may elapse from onset to rupture of the tympanic membrane. Chronic suppurative otitis media represents the residual stigmata of nonsuppurative or acute otitis media. It is these various residuals of chronic ear disease and its resultant hearing loss which otologists aim to prevent. By the early recognition and treatment of acute suppurative and nonsuppurative otitis media and the long-term follow-up until the ear stabilizes, we are able to prevent the resultant chronic ear disease, hearing loss, and residuals. Pain is seldom the presenting complaint in chronic suppurative otitis media, and the patient usually presents because of a purulent discharge from the ear canal or hearing loss.

Chronic suppurative otitis media is diagnosed by looking at the ear: There may be a tympanic membrane perforation, a cholesteatoma, or a marked retraction. Pus may or may not be present.

As will be seen in the following pages, the management of nonsuppurative otitis media and acute suppurative otitis media is relatively simple and very effective in preventing chronic ear disease and subsequent hearing loss. If treatment is delayed and if chronic ear disease ensues, the eradication of infection and restoration of hearing becomes a major problem inflicting additional emotional and physical hardship on the already handicapped patient and taxing the skill and patience of the otolaryngologist.

OTOLOGIC SURGERY

Ear surgery is indicated in patients with cleft palate for either acute or chronic nonsuppurative otitis media, or for acute or chronic suppurative otitis media, either active or inactive. All surgery upon the ear is performed utilizing the binocular operating microscope, thereby giving considerable magnification advantage over the naked eye. These operations may be considered under the following headings.

Myringotomy

Myringotomy is the incision of the pars tensa of the tympanic membrane to relieve exudate or pus in the tympanic cavity. In infants, anesthesia is not required. The arms and legs are confined by wrapping the infant in a sheet while an assistant holds the head steady. Working with the otologic operating microscope, an incision 2 to 3 mm in length is made in the posterior-inferior or inferior quadrant of the tympanic membrane. This position is chosen to prevent damage to the stapes bone or facial nerve. The incision generally heals extremely rapidly, first healing by coagulum and soon thereafter by healing of the pars tensa.

Myringotomy and Polyethylene Tube

Myringotomy is frequently indicated in nonsuppurative otitis media. Here prolonged ventilation of the middle ear may be required to allow time for the middle ear mucosa to return to normal. This is best accomplished by the insertion of a ventilation tube. These tubes may be of varying shapes and materials, but generally they remain in place for several months before being spontaneously extruded into the ear canal. Generally this extrusion from their resting position in the tympanic membrane is followed by rapid healing of the pars tensa of the tympanic membrane.

Simple Mastoidectomy

The simple mastoidectomy operation is designed to evacuate a coalescent abscess from within the mastoid process. While it is seldom required today, prior to the advent of sulfa and the antibiotics, it was the most frequently performed operation upon the temporal bones.

Following an episode of acute otitis media, a period of ten to fourteen days elapsed before acute coalescent mastoiditis developed. At this time, because most episodes of acute otitis media are treated with antibiotics, acute mastoiditis seldom develops. However, occasionally an apparently resistant strain of bacteria is present and this entity is encountered. When acute mastoiditis occurs in the cleft palate individual and does not respond to a wide myringotomy to drain the middle ear cavity of pus, and administration of intravenous antibiotics does not control the infection, then a simple mastoidectomy is required.

An incision is made behind the auricle and the mastoid bone is exposed. The outer layer of this bone is the cortex and is removed by a drill under the operating microscope. Soon, pus is encountered and allowed to escape from the incision. A drain is inserted, and antibiotic administration is continued. Usually, an uncomplicated postoperative course ensues.

Modified Radical and Radical Mastoidectomy

When chronic otitis media and cholesteatoma occurred in the patient with a cleft palate, the traditional operations would have been the modified radical and radical mastoidectomy. The choice of which operation would be performed depended on the location and extent of involvement of the middle ear and mastoid by cholesteatoma.

However, as pointed out so clearly by Sheehy,[6] the introduction of reconstructive techniques has brought about a gradual change in approach and a great reduction in the frequency of the performance of these operations. Both these operations entailed the exteriorization, rather than the removal, of cholesteatoma. The modified radical mastoidectomy is employed when the cholesteatoma is confined to the attic and mastoid portions of the temporal bone. The tympanic cavity is usually free of the disease, and the tympanic membrane and ossicles are usually preserved. Hearing may thus be quite good, both before and after the operation.

In the case of a patient whose middle ear and mastoid areas are filled with cholesteatoma, the radical mastoidectomy operation is performed. Here, to effect exteriorization of the cholesteatoma, frequently the tympanic membrane and ossicles are removed. Subsequently, there is frequently a significant conductive hearing loss on the operated site.

Both these operations usually result in a dry, safe ear.

Myringoplasty

This and the operations described hereafter required the individual to have an unobstructed eustachian tube. This is particularly important in the instance of the cleft palate individual.

Most ear infections subside, and the structures of the middle ear heal quickly. Infrequently, however, perforation of the eardrum may result. Myringoplasty is performed if a perforation of the tympanic membrane exists, but where there is no middle ear or mastoid infection and no disease of the middle ear bones. Various tissues usually taken from the patient are used to close the middle ear. A tissue frequently used at this time is fascia. This tissue heals the perforation with a high degree of consistency. Surgery may be performed under local or general anesthesia and usually entails only one to two days of hospitalization.

Tympanoplasty

An ear infection may cause damage to the ossicles (middle ear bones), in addition to causing a perforation in the eardrum. Tympanoplasty is the operation designed to repair both the tympanic membrane perforation and the ossicles of the sound-conducting mechanism. Various materials may be used to repair the tympanic membrane and reconstruct the ossicular chain. As mentioned earlier, fascia is a frequently used substitute for the tympanic membrane repair, while bone or cartilage are often used as ossicular substitutes. This surgery usually results in a sealed middle ear and often improves hearing. These operations are also performed either under local or general anesthesia and frequently require hospitalization for two to three days. The operation is performed either through the ear canal or from behind the ear.

Tympanoplasty with Mastoidectomy

Usually, chronic ear infection does not involve cholesteatoma. Almost always, the patients undergoing myringoplasty and tympanoplasty do not have cholesteatoma in addition to the tympanic membrane perforation and ossicular damage.

However, skin sometimes invades the middle ear and mastoid area, and a cholesteatoma is present. The cyst may be dry but, with time, frequently the cholesteatoma enlarges and results in a constant malodorous drainage. Should cholesteatoma be present, it must be removed at the time of eardrum and ossicular repair. This usually requires surgical entry into the mastoid as well as middle ear areas of the ear in order to gain enough exposure to permit complete removal of the disease.

Not infrequently, it is necessary to perform the operation in two stages. The first stage entails removal of the cholesteatoma and grafting the middle ear closed, and the second stage (usually performed eight to twelve months later) entails inspection for residual cholesteatoma and restoration of the hearing mechanism.

By utilizing the appropriate operation to suit the individual afflicted with chronic ear disease and cleft palate, a high degree of success may be anticipated in the elimination of the ear infection and the restoration of serviceable hearing to that individual.

REFERENCES

1. Paradise, J.L., Bluestone, C.D., and Felder, H.: The universality of otitis media in fifty infants with cleft palate. *Pediatrics, 44*:35-42, 1969.
2. Graham, M.D.: A longitudinal study of ear diseases and hearing loss in patients with cleft lips and palates. *Trans AAOO, 67*:213-222, 1963.
3. Schuknecht, H.F.: *Pathology of the Ear.* Cambridge, Harvard University Press, 1974, pg. 225.
4. Shambaugh, G.E., Jr.: *Surgery of the Ear.* Philadelphia, W. B. Saunders Company, 1967, pg. 217.
5. Glorig, A. and Gerwin, K.S.: *Otitis Media.* Springfield, Thomas, 1972, pg. 276.
6. Sheehy, J.L.: Surgery of Chronic Otitis Media. In *Otolaryngology,* Vol. II, Chapter 10. Hagerstown, Harper and Row, 1972.

—7—

COMMUNICATION PROBLEMS OF THE CHILD WITH CLEFT LIP AND CLEFT PALATE

JACQUELINE KEASTER

IN A STUDY[13] examining the birth records of all children born in a large county hospital over a fifteen-year period, it was found that 1 child in every 1,000 births was born with cleft palate. Of the children, 55 percent were male, and 25 percent had deformities other than cleft palates. The foregoing statistics are interesting, as they relate to the incidence of the condition, but do not imply the dire consequences to a child born with such a handicap in the development of acceptable speech and language. When a child with cleft lip and palate is born, the shock of the disfigurement to young parents, ill prepared for such a situation, may be so severe that it may cause them to abandon their newborn infant when the mother leaves the hospital. They cannot face the curiosity of relatives and friends, to say nothing of their own feelings of guilt over whether they may be responsible for having caused the condition. They may not even know that, when the child is two or three months old, he must have surgery to close his lip; that when he is from twelve to eighteen months old, he will need to have a second operation to close his palate. If there is sufficient tissue and the musculature is properly developed, he may learn to speak with normal voice quality and with articulation free of the stigmata of cleft palate.

In a review of the histories of 612 children whose palates had been repaired and who had not received routine speech therapy or intensive postoperative follow-up, it was found[11] that 39.7 percent had normal speech. This tends to suggest that about 60 percent of children born with cleft lip and palate go through much more than two surgical procedures in order to ensure an adequate mechanism for the development of speech that does not call attention to itself because of its hypernasal quality and defective articulation. Jim is a case in point:

> He is now twelve and in junior high school. He was born with a bilateral cleft in the posterior two thirds of his soft palate. He did not have a cleft lip. His palate was operated for the first time when he was thirteen months old. On the day of surgery, it was noted that he had serous otitis media and that both tympanic cavities were filled with fluid. Because of his age, his hearing was not tested. He had an uneventful recovery from the surgical procedure and was not seen again until he was six years of age. At that time, the complaint was *rhinolalia aperta,* or hypernasality. Apparently there had not been sufficient tissue available when the palate was operated to effect a closure at the nasopharynx. In an effort to provide more tissue, a pharyngeal flap procedure was carried out. It was not successful, and a year later adhesions were removed surgically and a prosthesis was fitted. When this was completed, Jim's speech was markedly improved. Shortly afterward, a conductive hearing loss of about 35 dB bilateral was noted, a condition that may have existed to a greater or lesser extent from infancy. A question arose concerning whether the prosthesis might be impinging upon the orifice of the eustachian tube irritating the hearing loss. Adjustments were made and an improvement in hearing was noted. When last seen, his threshold for pure tones in his better ear was 15 dB. His speech and language were excellent. His only concern was whether he could continue to wear the appliance during the course of orthodontic treatment that was about to begin.

Such a series of procedures as Jim went through in order to attain an adequate mechanism for the development of good speech and language is not unusual for a child born with cleft palate. Some go through much more and may attain something less than adequate results because there was so little to work with.

George von Bekesy, who contributed greatly to our understanding of how the ear works, was once heard to say, "Hearing is awful complicated." The same might be said of the communication problems of the child born with cleft lip and palate or cleft palate alone. He may experience some delay in the onset of speech and language, his voice quality may be hypernasal, and he may have a sufficient number of articulation errors to render his speech all but unintelligible. More importantly, the problems are frequently made more complex because of the reactions of parents, family members, and friends over his disfigurement if he has a cleft lip and sometimes over his inability to nurse in the normal manner because of the hole in his palate. Either or both conditions tend to affect the quality of mothering that he may receive. McCarthy[15] has pointed out:

> The Mother is normally the child's first language teacher in our culture, and it is she who furnishes the example for the baby to imitate. It is her voice that he echoes back in his babbling and her smile and fondling which most often elicit his cooing and other prelinguistic utterances. Studies indicate that it is not merely this quantitative aspect of the mother-child relationship which is important but that the quality of that relationship has a significant influence on the acquisition of language.

In the foregoing quotation, the author was referring to the acquisition of language in the normal child. One can only suppose that the quantity and quality of mothering is even more important in the language development of the child with cleft lip and cleft palate. The first task of the professional people involved is in helping his family to understand and to accept him as a person in spite of all of his problems.

> One is reminded of a preschooler and his mother who once came a long distance once each week for speech therapy. Bill was the youngest of four boys and the only one in the family with any kind of handicapping condition. Each time he came for speech therapy, his mother took the opportunity to provide a day just for him when they could do what he enjoyed most without interference from the older brothers. They both enjoyed the time together tremendously. This was only one of the thoughtful ways that Bill was made to feel that he was special. In spite of a deeply scarred upper lip and some marked nasal emission. he was friendly and outgoing with the affect of a little boy who was indeed much loved. It was his charming manner one noticed rather this his imperfections in speech and appearance. His voice quality was nasal, his articulation was faulty, but his language development was superior for his age.

In a study[22] of language skills of forty children with cleft lip and palate but with normal hearing, it was found that, as a group, the children studied had superior recognition vocabularies, but a retarded amount of verbal output and vocabulary usage. It was believed that the findings were possibly related to the child's evaluation of himself and of his speech, a situation that would appear to be related not only to the quantity but the quality of the mothering that had been received.

In assessing the speech and language of a young child with cleft palate, it is well to remember that many children under the age of five with no palatal deformity have language that is infantile in structure with articulation patterns that make speech almost unintelligible, unless one listens very carefully. Such speech problems result from a multiplicity of factors — social, psychological, and physical — which may also operate in affecting the speech and language development in the child with cleft palate. He, like his counterpart with normal palatal structures, may be born into a family where there is limited speech stimulation.

> A story[3] is told of a five-year-old child, reared on a farm in Iowa, who presented at a University Speech Clinic with a complaint of retarded speech and language. He was proved to be normal mentally and physically, but most of his waking hours from the age of two were spent with an aged grandmother who rarely spoke. His parents were out in the fields. His only companion was his pet dog whose brand of affection did not include speech.

Such a situation is, perhaps, extreme, but serves to illustrate the need for verbal stimulation in the child with or without cleft palate, if speech is to be learned at the expected age. Speech learning is basically an imitative process, and there must be a pattern to follow.

Children born with cleft lip and cleft palate, like all children, follow the normal curve in intelligence. Some are very bright, some very dull, and the majority fall within the normal range. It is well known that children whose intelligence is at the lower end of the curve, with or without palatal deformities, are likely to have speech that is slow to develop, immature in language structure, with poor articulation. In extreme cases, he may never learn to communicate verbally. One study[5] of 122 children born with cleft palate found that 14 had developed no words at two years and three months, of age and no phrases by three years. Of the 14, 9 were below average in intelligence, 3 of the 9 were mentally defective, and 4 were found to have bilateral hearing losses.

It is often observed that a bright child with a poorly functioning mechanism may have much more normal speech and language than a child not so bright whose palatal structures are more nearly normal. The bright child may be more able to compensate for his structural inadequacies, or he may just have more to say and take more care about the way he says it.

Many children without cleft palate have delayed and often defective speech and language as a result of congenital or acquired sensorineural hearing loss of varying degree. Such losses are, in most cases, permanent and require the use of a hearing aid for amelioration. There have been cases cited in the literature of children with cleft palate who also have sensorineural hearing losses, but such instances are comparatively rare. One study[21] of 401 children with cleft palate cited such cases, all the result of disease in early infancy. Another study[20] cited one child in a group of thirty consecutive cases with a sensorineural loss thought to have been congenital.

Children with cleft palate, however, are known to have more middle ear disease and, as a consequence, more conductive hearing losses than do children without the palatal deformity. In reviewing the literature on the incidence of hearing loss in such children, it becomes obvious that the percentages vary greatly depending upon the definition of hearing loss being used.[9,23] A medically significant loss, one that indicates to the otologist the possible presence of ear pathology, must be judged by a different set of criteria from that of an educationally or socially significant loss which, to the teacher or speech and hearing specialist, may be an indication for special handling in the classroom.

In a study[18] of fifty infants with cleft palate twenty months of age or younger, it was found that all had bilateral secretory or supporative otitis media. In a comparable group of one hundred infants without cleft palates, it was found that only 22 percent had ear disease. The authors say that, because a conductive hearing loss of appreciable degree is likely to accompany such a condition, it seems reasonable to suppose that some of the later communication problems typical of children with cleft palate may be attributable to early hearing losses, especially if the condition causing them is untreated. A case in point is that of Michael.

He was born on December 10, 1969, with a cleft lip and palate. His lip was repaired when he was seven months old and his palate when he was nineteen months. When he was two years of age, he was brought to a Children's Hospital Emergency Clinic with an acute otitis media in the left ear with a chronic otitis media in the right. The condition was treated medically and a follow-up appointment given for Ear, Nose and Throat Clinic. The appointment was not kept, even after social service intervention. One can only assume that when the earache stopped, Michael's family thought there was no longer a problem so they did not keep the appointment. Three months later the ear flared up again, and this time he was brought to the Ear, Nose and Throat Clinic. He had bilateral otitis media that was treated medically and a myringotomy with polyethylene tube was scheduled. His hearing was tested using conditioned orientation reflex audiometry, with warbled tones in a sound field. He responded to the following:

250	500	1000	2000	4000
60	60	50	40	40

He responded to voice and music at 60 dB. This was considered to be a minimum estimate of his hearing acuity. Four subsequent appointments for hearing reevaluation were failed. In the meantime, his mother refused to permit the otologist to perform the myringotomy. Ten months later his hearing was retested. He was now almost four years old. It was possible to obtain a speech reception threshold using pictures of common objects at 50 dB. His responses to pure tones were roughly comparable to those on the previous test. Michael could not be tested using play audiometry, because of his immaturity. Approximately eight months later, he returned to the Ear, Nose and Throat Clinic, this time with bilateral otitis media and a complaint by his mother that he did not hear unless spoken to in a loud voice. When his hearing was tested, it was found that his speech reception threshold, using common objects, was 40 dB. Play audiometry was again attempted. A pure tone audiogram was obtained that was considered reliable using both air– and bone-conducted sound. Bone conduction was relatively normal with air conduction, as had been suggested by previous tests.

Michael is a personable little boy with poorly developed speech and language due in part to a hearing loss of at least 40 dB since he was an infant. There has been a paucity of real language stimulation in the home. His mother has never really understood the relationship between the ear pathology represented to her by earaches and his very apparent hearing loss. She is beginning to realize that his speech and language development are markedly delayed. With this realization, she has now given her consent for an otologic procedure that should improve his hearing before the loss becomes permanent. He can then have help in the development of speech and language before entering school.

Studies[7,14,20,23] concerning hearing loss in children with cleft palate have all suggested that the incidence is far higher than in children without a palatal deformity. There is evidence to suggest that such losses fluctuate and become less severe as the child matures.[6] Because of the fact that ear pathology has been found in young infants with cleft palate, it is important that the hearing of all such infants be tested as soon as they are mature enough to respond to some sort of audiometry. Obviously, the younger the child, the less definitive the test results, but it is possible to get an indication of the presence or absence of hearing loss in a baby as young as eight to ten months, an age when he is beginning to do a great deal of babbling and imitating of the speech sounds around him. By the time a child is three years old, it is frequently possible to test his hearing by both air and bone conduction, using play audiometry and modified speech threshold testing as a validating measure. The latter test has considerable value as an indication of how handicapping a hearing loss may be at any given time to any child but especially to one with cleft palate.

Sometimes the known presence of ear pathology with a mild hearing loss may be overinterpreted as a deterrent to speech and language development when, at the same time, other factors bearing consideration are ignored. The child being examined may be slow in all areas of development, or he may have had limited speech stimulation at a time when speech ordinarily develops. The mild hearing loss may not be, in his case, "a difference that makes a difference."

On the other hand, a hearing loss of 30 dB or greater in the better ear can be a severe deterrent in the development of speech and language, especially if it occurs in the preschool years. A child with such a loss may also have real problems in following what is being said to him if the speaker is at any distance away or is not facing him. In order to help him to understand more easily, he may need some lipreading instruction. If he is in school, he will certainly need advantageous seating in the classroom, that is, a spot where he is best able to hear instructions given by his teacher and the give-and-take of discussion between the teacher and his fellow students. In most such cases, a hearing aid will not be necessary because of the transitory nature of the hearing loss.

It has been estimated[13] that about 25 percent of children born with cleft lip and cleft palate have other congenital anomalies. One writer[2] has suggested the possibility of problems in the development of the tongue musculature accounting for some of the pronounced articulatory defects unrelated to palatal function occurring with more than coincidental frequency. It has been suggested that children crippled in the palate may also be crippled in the tongue. When articulation problems persist in spite of great effort to effect a change, consideration should be given to the possibility of a malformation in the tongue preventing the child from attaining more nearly normal articulation.

Another more obvious related anomaly is atresia of the external auditory canal, sometimes in one ear and other times in both. Such an obstruction will, in most instances, result in a hearing loss by air conduction of 45 to 50 dB in all frequencies. If the problem is confined to the external ear, responses should be within the normal range to bone conduction. If the condition exists in only one ear, it should not affect speech development or prevent the child's following verbal directions given at normal levels. But if the atresia is bilateral and it can be demonstrated audiometrically that he has a normally functioning inner ear, he should be fitted with a hearing aid with a bone conduction receiver. Many children under the age of two years have been fitted with such a device to be used until they were old enough for a surgical procedure to open the canal. With relatively normal bone conduction, such children learn speech and language without undue delay if there are no other deterring factors.

In summary, it may be said that about 60 percent of children born with cleft lip and cleft palate will have problems in learning to communicate verbally. Some may suffer from the rejection of parents and relatives, others may have hearing losses that make self-monitoring difficult, while others may have insufficient palatal tissue to effect a proper closure at the nasopharynx. Many will undergo a number of surgical procedures, long periods of orthodontic treatment and, sometimes, a prosthesis and long hours of speech therapy before they attain acceptable speech and language.

REFERENCES

1. Backus, O.L.: Children with cleft palate and cleft lip. In Johnson and Wendell (Ed.): *Speech Problems of Children,* New York, Grune & Stratton, 1950, p. 117.
2. Berry, M.F.: Lingual anomolies associated with palatal clefts. *Speech Hear Disord, 14*(4):359, 1949.
3. Brown, S.F.: Cleft palate. In Johnson and Wendell (Ed.): *Speech Handicapped School Children,* 2nd ed., New York, Harper & Bros., 1956, p. 330.
4. Counihan, Donald T.: Articulation skills of adolescents and adults with cleft palates. *J Speech, Hear Disord, 25*(#2):181, May 1960.
5. Drillien, C.M., Ingram, T.T.S., and Wilkinson, E.M.: *The Causes and Natural History of Children with Cleft Palates.* Baltimore, The Williams & Wilkins Co., 1966, p. 155.
6. Goetzinger, C.P.: A study of hearing level and auditory discrimination in cleft palate adults. *Cleft Pal Bull, 10:*65, 1960.
7. Graham, M.D.: A longitudinal study of ear disease and hearing loss in patients with cleft lips and palates. *Annals of Otol Rhinol Laryngol, 73:*34, 1964.
8. Hahn, E.: Speech therapy for the pre-school cleft palate child. *J Speech Hear Disord, 23:*605, Nov. 1957.
9. Hayes, C.S.: Audiologic Problems Associated with Cleft Palate. *Proceedings of the Conference: Communicative Problems in Cleft Palate ASHA Reports,* April, 1965, p. 83.
10. Koepp-Baker, H.: Speech problems of the person with cleft lip and cleft palate. In Travis, L.E. (Ed.): *Handbook of Speech Pathology.* New York, Appleton-Century-Crofts, 1957, p. 597.
11. Lindsay, W.K., LeMesurier, M.D., and Farmer, A.W.: A study of the

speech results of a large series of cleft palate patients. *Plast Reconstr Surg, 29*(#3):273, March 1962.
12. Lis, E.F., Pruzansky, S., Koepp-Baker, H., and Kobes, H.R.: Cleft lip and cleft palate. *Pediatr Clin North Am,* 995, Nov. 1956.
13. Lutz, K.R. and Moor, F.B.: A study of factors in the occurrence of cleft palate. *J Speech Hear Disord, 20*(#3):271, Sept. 1955.
14. Masters, F.W., Bingham, H.G., and Robinson, D.W.: The prevention and treatment of hearing loss in the cleft palate child. *Plast Reconstr Surg, 25*:503, 1960.
15. McCarthy, D.: Language disorders and parent-child relationships. *J Speech Hear Disord, 19*(#4):514, Dec. 1954.
16. Millard, R.D.: Wide and/or short cleft palate. *Plast Reconstr Surg, 29:* 40, Jan. 1965.
17. Morris, H.L.: Communication skills of children with cleft lips and palates. *J Speech Hear Res, 5*(#1):79, March 1962.
18. Paradise, J.L., Bluestone, C., and Felder, H.: The university of otitis media in 50 infants with cleft palate, *Pediatrics, 44:*(#1):35, July 1969.
19. Powers, G.R.: Cinefluorographic investigation of articulatory movements of selected individuals with cleft palate. *J Speech & Hear Res, 5*(#1):59, Mar. 1962.
20. Sataloff, J and Fraser, M.: Hearing loss in children with cleft palate, *Arch Otol, 55*:61, 1952.
21. Skolnik, E.M.: Otologic evaluation of cleft palate patients. *Laryngoscope, 68* (Pt. 2):1908, 1958.
22. Spriestersbach, D.C., Darley, F., and Morris, H.: Language skills in children with cleft palate. *J Speech Hear Res, 1*(#3):279, Sept. 1958.
23. Spriestersbach, D.C., Lierle, D.M., Moll, K.L., and Prather, W.F.: Hearing loss in children with cleft palates. *Plast Reconstr Surg, 30:*336, Sept. 1962.
24. Vini, C. and Alan, R.: Clinical evaluation of cleft palate patients and their speech. *Plast Reconstr Surg, 25:*496, 1960.
25. Williams, H.B. and Woolhouse, F.M.: Comparison of speech improvement in cases of cleft palate after two methods of pharyngoplasty. *Plast Reconstr Surg, 30:*36, July 1962.

8

HEARING IMPAIRMENT AND LANGUAGE LEARNING DISORDERS*

DANIEL LING, PH.D.†

THIS CHAPTER CONSISTS of three major parts. First, a sample survey is reported which indicates characteristics common to many children with cleft palate. Second, the literature relating to various factors affecting language learning in cleft palate children is reviewed. Finally, hearing loss as a major contributing factor is discussed, and various means of providing preventative and remedial treatment for language learning problems arising from hearing loss are presented. Throughout the chapter, emphasis is placed upon factors associated with learning problems common to the whole range of children who may be seen in a cleft palate clinic, rather than on individual differences in relation to the type or extent of cleft palate anomaly.

INTRODUCTION

Poor hearing in childhood is known to lead to difficulties, not just in school subjects, but in total personal-social development.

*The preparation of this chapter was supported by Canadian Health Grant 604-7-725.

†I am most grateful to Sally Jo Naish who helped extensively both in the literature search and by typing the manuscript and to Janet Ashdown who assisted in collating the data for the sample survey collected by Dr. W.W. Tidmarsh and the cleft palate team of the Montreal Children's Hospital. Thanks are due to my colleagues on the teaching staff of the McGill School of Human Communication Disorders who suggested revisions to the initial draft.

Many children with cleft palate are known to have some degree of hearing impairment, and in this chapter the extent to which hearing may be impaired and how cleft palate, hearing impairment, or both may affect intellectual characteristics, personality, and language skills are explored.

In all special groups, a wide range of individual differences is found, both in the severity of the primary abnormality and the extent of associated disorders. The importance of these two types of individual differences cannot be overemphasised, for they must be constantly borne in mind by the clinician whose work is to evaluate and cater to the needs of individuals.

SAMPLE SURVEY

As a first step towards writing this chapter, data was collected on ninety-two of the children seen by the cleft palate team at the Montreal Children's Hospital. This sample comprised sixty males and thirty-two females ranging in age from infant to sixteen years. The children were selected only on the basis of accessibility; only those living within the Greater Montreal area were included. The sample, therefore, represented a wide range of children with cleft palate and associated anomalies. Only four of the sample had average unilateral hearing loss over the frequencies 250 to 4000 Hz in excess of 30 dB (ISO), whereas sixteen had bilateral hearing loss of equivalent severity. Some thirty-five children had average hearing levels better than 10 dB (ISO). Thus, fifty-seven children, almost two thirds of the sample, had some degree of hearing loss. In all cases, this was of the conductive type arising from middle ear pathology. Of the total sample, forty-nine had at some time received specific medical or surgical treatment for ear disease, ten at or below two years, twenty-seven at three to four years, and eleven of the remaining twelve at five to six years of age. The remaining child first received otological treatment at the age of twelve. While most were treated fairly early in life, the treatment was not immediately or permanently effective. Records indicated that hearing loss tended to fluctuate from one audiometric examination to the next, although there was a tendency for hearing loss to be less severe among the older than among the younger children. This sample, then, demonstrated a high proportion of diagnosed hearing loss which could have potentially caused learning difficulties.

Intelligence (WISC or Stanford-Binet) tests had been administered to thirty of the ninety-two children referred for testing on account of additional problems, such as hyperactivity, poor attention, and learning disorders. All thirteen children who had been tested with the WISC obtained poorer scores on the verbal than on the performance scale. Otherwise, the results were unremarkable.

Speech had been rated as slightly deviant in fifty-four of the children and markedly deviant in ten others. In forty-three of the sixty-four children who had received speech therapy, hearing loss averaging 20 dB or more was present over the frequencies 250 to 4000 Hz. Of the sixty-four children, twenty-six were considered to have language deficits, eight of whom, all with marked hearing loss, were considered to have more than slight problems. The hearing, psychological, and language characteristics of this sample appear to be fairly typical, as indicated by numerous studies reported in the literature reviewed and discussed below.

HEARING, PSYCHOLOGICAL, AND LANGUAGE CHARACTERISTICS

Hearing Impairment

As Bluestone (*see* Chapter 4) has demonstrated, hearing impairment is commonly associated with cleft palate. The prevalence and extent of such hearing impairment vary in relation to age, the nature of the cleft palate lesions, the age of the child at the time of corrective oral surgery, the provision of otological treatment, and of course, the criteria set for classifying a child as hearing impaired.[1-6] Hayes[7] has proposed that hearing loss in children with cleft palate is of educational significance if it averages 20 dB (ISO?) over the frequency range 500 to 2000 Hz. The problem with attempting to define educational significance in such terms is that it excludes other variables, such as the age of the child, known to be of considerable importance. Further, such a definition assumes the hearing loss to be a relatively stable entity. Age is an important variable, because early infancy appears to be the optimal period for first language acquisition. Hearing impairment can, therefore, be expected to influence the development of speech communication skills more adversely if it is present in and from early infancy than if its onset occurs at a later stage. The assumption that conductive hearing loss in cleft palate children may be regarded as stable is unacceptable. Their hearing levels are known to vary considerably not only with eustachian tube function from day to day,[5] but from one month to the next,[8] over the course of several years. In this latter regard, it has been noted that children with cleft palate over six years of age tend to have less hearing loss than those under that age.[3] Nevertheless, the 20 dB hearing level that Hayes suggests as cause for educational concern has much to recommend it. Although most audiometric screening tests in schools are administered at or about 25 dB (ISO), overall hearing loss in children at a 20 dB level has frequently been shown to be associated with poor speech discrimination and educational deficits.[9-14] In some cases, deficits associated with such a slight loss may have accumulated throughout a long history of more severe impairment, which has ameliorated with time. In other cases, there may be genuine difficulty in learning speech discrimination skills through an auditory mechanism fluctuating between adequacy and inadequacy from day to day, due to the presence of active middle ear disease. That such ear disease may be observed otoscopically in children whose hearing is well within normal limits has been shown in studies of two fairly large school populations.[15,16]

Intellectual Characteristics

The literature on intelligence in children with cleft palate is meagre, but indicates that, in general estimates, their intelligence tends to be somewhat lower than a normal population. While some children with cleft palate have superior intellectual abilities, more are below than above average.

Among the first to study the problem were Billig[17] in the United States and Illingworth and Birch[18] in England. In both studies, the mean intelligence of the children on a variety of tests was found to be in the low average range. Illingworth and Birch suggested that the poorer intellectual ability found might be due to genetic selection, arising from forbears with hare lip and cleft palate having accepted "mates of inferior social status and appearance." Some support for this suggestion was provided by Munson and May,[19] who found not only that there was a significantly larger number of children with cleft palates below than above average intelligence, but that the socioeconomic status of the parents of their 132 subjects, all drawn from Pennsylvania, was significantly poorer than the state norm. Lewis,[20] however, on the basis of findings in a survey of 548 subjects and their families, stated that "the anomaly (of cleft palate) itself, or related factors, have a more significant bearing on the difference in mean IQ than the (socio-economic status of the) family."

The first study to demonstrate that intelligence test results among cleft palate children were associated with hearing loss was undertaken in 1954.[21] In this study Means and Irvin, using the Stanford-Binet test, found that among those with hearing loss, mean intelligence was significantly lower than normal, whereas among those with hearing levels better than 25 dB it was not. In later studies,[22-24] which have used control groups of siblings or children matched in socioeconomic status, mean performance quotients obtained on the Wechsler Scale have been slightly, but significantly, below the norms for the test (which supports the notion of a selective, genetic factor) and mean verbal quotients of the cleft palate subjects have been significantly poorer than their performance quotients. This latter discrepancy, though amounting to less than ten points on the Wechsler Scale, indicates that speech and hearing problems, perhaps hearing loss in particular, may contribute more than most other factors to the depressed verbal intelligence scores and learning difficulties experienced by children with cleft palate. If this is so, then preventative and remedial measures, as discussed later, could ameliorate this situation.

Personality Characteristics

Most research over several decades has failed to demonstrate any marked personality defects common to children with cleft palates.[22] This is rather surprising, since as Clifford[25] points out, it is commonly assumed that disfigurement (as with cleft lip), feeding difficulties, hospitalization as an infant, surgical attention to the face and/or mouth, speech defects, and parental difficulty in accepting a child with a physical defect are all adverse conditions, any one of which might lead to an evident personality disorder. However, clinicians seldom find it necessary to refer a child with cleft palate for psychiatric help,[26] and as Birch[27] reported in 1952, of 600 children rated as severely maladjusted in the Pittsburgh public schools, not one was a child with cleft palate.

More recently, one experimental study[28] has shown that there were no significant differences in scores on the Rogers Personal Adjustment Inventory among three groups of boys having cleft lip and cleft palate, cleft palate only, and no known physical handicap. Another study,[29] in which projective tests were employed with cleft palate children and their siblings, revealed fewer differences than would have been expected by chance. It has also been shown[30] that a group of children with cleft palate behaved similarly to their peers in relation to dropping out or staying in high school.

Not all studies have yielded data indicating completely normal personal-social development. One has indicated that children with cleft palate have impaired ability to think creatively,[31] and another[32] that older subjects with cleft palate (aged fifteen to thirty-five years) are less well adapted than a normal control group in high school education, occupational training, family life, and participation in social activities. The findings in this latter study would not have been predicted from the work of Goodstein,[23] who found scores on the Vineland Social Maturity Scale, though depressed with cleft palate children under five years, to be less so as age increased. On the basis of several studies, McWilliams[33] considers children with cleft palate to be somewhat passive, compliant, and self-effacing. If these are genuine group characteristics, then it is not surprising that so few are regarded as having personality problems. Hostile and aggressive behaviors are much more readily noticed and probably constitute a greater obstacle to learning. The evidence for slight personality disorders in this group is, nevertheless, not too convincing. Severe personality disorders are quite atypical. Most children with cleft palate appear to be essentially well adjusted, with no more personality problems than the "children next door."

Language Skills

There is a considerable body of evidence that children with cleft palate tend to be retarded in a wide variety of language skills.[34] There are many possible reasons why this might be so. As a group, mean intelligence, socioeconomic background and speech and hearing skills have, as mentioned above, been found to be somewhat depressed. Additionally, since surgery involving inpatient care is involved, hospitalization may be a contributing factor. Parent's attitudes, as well as those of others in the environment, may also lead to a reduced verbal experience. Careful evaluation of the literature does not suggest that the general picture of language retardation is an artifact arising, for example, from selective sampling of the type that might bias results. Certainly, selective sampling has been employed in many studies, but children who have been excluded — such as those with marked hearing loss, or a history of extensive hospitalization — would have been likely to present a greater degree of language deficit.

Measures of language ability employed in various studies include the extent of babbling, age the first word was spoken, use of jargon, age the first sentences were employed, mean length of response, structural complexity, Mecham's Verbal Language Development Scale, the Language Ability Test (comprised of selected verbal items from a number of intelligence tests), the Ammons Full-Range Picture Vocabulary Test, the Peabody Picture Vocabulary Test, and the Illinois Test of Psycholinguistic Abilities. Babbling tends to be delayed, as does the use of first words, jargon, and first sentences.[35] With one exception,[36] vocabulary recognition has been found to be poorer than normal,[37-40] and vocabulary usage poorer than vocabulary recognition.[38] In one of these studies,[37] some degree of retardation was found among 107 subjects aged two to fifteen years on eleven language measures. In another,[39] the Illinois Test of Psycholinguistic Abilities was administered to 136 children and scores compared to the standardization data at each of six age levels (three to eight years, inclusive). A general depression on all nine subtests was found. There was a tendency for language weaknesses to become more marked as age increased, a finding common to at least one other study.[40] Whether such linguistic weaknesses persist into adult life has not yet been established. Perhaps adequate education may overcome them, a possibility suggested by a study of written language of elementary school children,[41] in which no differences between a cleft palate group and normal controls were found.

It does not seem likely that generally poor intelligence can entirely explain the overall language deficits noted, since such deficits have also been found among many children with cleft palate having better than average intelligence. While Templin,[42] among others, has shown socioeconomic status and language skills to be related in normal children drawn from an urban community, studies with cleft palate children, most from mixed (urban and rural) communities, have failed to show any notable relationship of this type. Many writers have speculated on the possible reasons for failing to find language skills to be better in subjects who come from homes which rate highly on the socioeconomic scale, but no research based on such speculation has been undertaken. A similar situation exists in relation to speech. The speech of children with cleft palate is, with certain exceptions, generally abnormal.[43] The relationships between poor speech skills and language deficits is an intriguing area for speculation, theory, and research. In fact, it has generated almost none of these. Speculation in the literature to date[34,37,44] is very limited. One suggestion is that children finding it difficult to express themselves in intelligible speech retreat to the persistent use of simple language forms, but this would not explain the problems these children have in vocabulary acquisition and usage. Philips and Harrison,[40] however, consider that retardation at all levels might stem from parental rejection of distorted speech patterns, resulting in deprivation of normal feedback and reinforcement. They report observations which lend support to this hypothesis. Speculation has not extended even to the possibility of support for the motor theory of speech perception[45] and linguistic analysis of the type undertaken by Menyuk,[46] or studies of transformational structures of the type suggested by Lee and Canter[47] have not been published on children with cleft palate. Yet, since there does appear to be a relationship between poor speech skills and language deficits in these children,[37] the problem should obviously receive more attention. Of course, the association may not be entirely causal, since, for example, hearing loss (which itself may be determined by the nature of the cleft) can result in both speech and language deficits. That the degree of hearing loss can affect the intelligibility of speech among cleft palate children has been demonstrated.[48] That it can adversely affect language development in children with cleft palate has also been shown,[49] even when children with hearing levels above 30 dB (ASA) have been excluded from the majority of studies.

With the exception of duration of hospitalization,[49] no other possible factor has been shown to account for the overall language deficit commonly found in children with cleft palate. Numerous articles reviewed by McWilliams[26] and Pannbacker[34] have emphasized the possible effects on language skills of parental adjustment, perhaps influenced by the time at which the cleft is discovered, reaction to the birth of a defective child, concern about appearance, feeding, surgical measures, financial considerations, and reactions of family and friends. In only one study, however, has the adjustment of parents of cleft palate children been shown to differ significantly from that of a normal group.[50] Strangely enough, parents of older, but not younger, cleft palate children were found to be the more poorly adjusted. If this finding has general validity, then it speaks poorly for the overall quality of management provided for the cleft palate child. The data pointing to general language deficits also suggest that speech problems, which are relatively easy to identify, tend to be given attention by the therapist to the exclusion of the less obvious, but vital, need of the child to develop optimum linguistic competency. That the therapist must routinely deal with more than the speech aspects of cleft palate children's problems has been strongly suggested by Smith and McWilliams.[51] The final section of this chapter, in addition to outlining the principles of hearing for speech, provides some suggestions in this regard.

HEARING IMPAIRMENT, SPEECH RECEPTION, AND LANGUAGE DEVELOPMENT

The extent to which hearing loss can hinder speech reception depends not only on the type and degree of hearing impairment, but also on the power and integrity of the speech signal. Sensorineural hearing loss probably occurs no more frequently among cleft palate children than it does in a normal population, whereas conductive hearing impairment is a pervasive problem. Our concern here, therefore, is mainly with conductive hearing impairment.

Conductive impairment tends to reduce sensitivity more or less equally across the whole frequency range of hearing. Such a hearing loss can be produced simply by plugging the external ear canal. In fact, to do just this and experiment with speech perception would give the reader first hand experience of the hearing problem faced by many cleft palate children. The experiment, to be realistic, would have to be carried out in a child's home, his school, where children play, and, of course, the extent of hearing loss would have to be varied. One thing the reader would not be able to simulate by such a procedure would be the general feeling of malaise that often accompanies persistent middle ear infection, though empathy might compensate for this. Of course, coming to such a situation with extensive language skills, the reader would also find it hard to appreciate how much more impaired the child would be because his restricted experience of communication.

Hearing Loss and Speech

Hearing loss, as charted on an audiogram, shows the intensity level (in dB) at which the subject can just detect the presence of pure tones at frequencies ranging from 125 to 8000 Hz. This range represents the approximate frequency range of speech. The fundamental (larynx tone) of a male voice often falls around 125 Hz, and the highest components of a fricative sound, such as /s/, may occur up to about 8000 Hz. Most speech sounds fall in the middle of this range, from about 500 to 2000 Hz. Zero dB on the audiogram represents the threshold levels for pure tones of each frequency of the average, normally hearing young adult. Children's threshold hearing levels may be better than these.[15]

Speech sounds cannot be accurately represented by points on an audiogram because of their complexity. Each speech sound has characteristic components which can be approximately specified in terms of frequency, intensity, and time; these components vary from speaker to speaker, in relation to the context and according to the overall intensity of the speech. For example, an adult female's voice is higher than that of a male speaker's, and a child's voice may be higher still; the frequency range of a /t/ changes in accordance with the vowel preceding or following it. In addition, Speakers not only vary the intensity of their voices, but the intensity of sound decreases with distance. Nevertheless, to represent average frequencies and intensities of certain sounds on an audiogram can be helpful in illustrating the effect of hearing loss on speech reception.

The audiogram in Figure 8-1 shows the frequency and intensity of five sounds spoken by the writer at a distance of two yards from the microphone of an analysing device. The sounds are /u/ as in wh*o*, /a/ as in f*a*ther, /i/ as in k*ey*, /ʃ/ as in *sh*oe, and /s/ as in *s*it.

Only the two lower formants (peaks of resonance) of the three vowels have been included. Inspection of this figure shows that a child with an overall hearing loss of 35 dB would miss some of these five sounds and, of course, some of the thirty or so other speech sounds which share this frequency range and are of much the same intensity. Remember that these sounds were spoken at a distance of only 2 yards. Had they been spoken closer to the microphone (listener), they would have been louder, and from further away, quieter.

Sound decreases in intensity by about 6 dB with every dou-

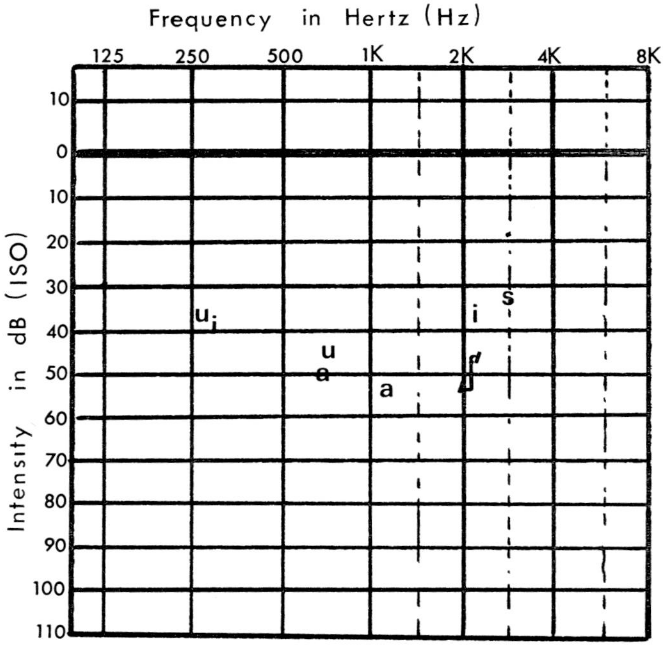

Figure 8-1. Audiogram showing hearing levels of the three vowels /a/, /u/, and /i/, and the consonants /ʃ/ and /s/ generated by the writer speaking naturally at a distance of 2 yards from the microphone of an analysing device.

bling of distance, except when it is reflected from surrounding hard surfaces. Thus, if the speaker does not raise his voice level, the intensity of these sounds at a distance of 4 yards would measure about 6 dB less and at 8 yards about 12 dB less. By subtracting 12 dB from each sound on the audiogram, it becomes clear that the /s/ would not then be heard at 8 yards by the child with a 25 dB hearing loss, and the remaining sounds would be barely audible. To be sure, most speech is directed to a child at a distance of less than 8 yards, but much incidental, ongoing speech in a child's environment occurs at greater distances, and children do not learn entirely from speech directed to them. Further, normally hearing children do not listen near threshold, where the sounds may be audible but not identifiable. They not only hear sounds over much greater distances than the child with a mild hearing loss, but hear them loud enough to ensure their identification. A reserve of hearing appears to be necessary for language learning. Even adults, listening to a radio program in a second language in which they are not perfectly fluent, usually increase the volume to a level well above that required to understand their mother tongue. Thus, a hearing loss which constitutes no serious problem to an adult may be devastating to a child in the process of language acquisition.

There are three ways to increase the intensity of speech to the level required by the child with hearing impairment: talking louder, talking closer to the child, and using some form of amplification. Talking louder is clearly undesirable and may lead to the speaker developing a voice disorder. The objective is to overcome one communication deficit, not to create another. Talking closer to the child is far more effective than most people imagine. Earlier it was explained that sound level drops by about 6 dB each time the distance is doubled. Conversely, it increases by 6 dB each time distance is halved. Thus by speaking from a distance of 1 yard rather than 2, one gains 6 dB, and at 18 inches rather than 2 yards, 12 dB. As hearing problems are most likely to occur in early infancy among cleft palate children and, as early infancy is the optimal period for language development, training parents to handle, play with, and read to their young children within touching distance could avoid many of the problems caused by hearing loss. Many activities with the young child (feeding, changing, etc.) demand handling. Many more such activities can be contrived so that speech reaches the young child at an appropriate level.

A tape recorder may be used to demonstrate the effect of distance on speech levels to parents and teachers. By adjusting the input level meter to peak at zero when speaking some 6 inches or so from the microphone, and then moving back to 12 inches, 2 feet, 4 feet, and 8 feet, the successive drop of about 6 dB with increasing distance is heard with dramatic clarity. The reader is strongly urged to include this demonstration in counselling teachers, parents, or students who will be professionally concerned with patients having problems in hearing for speech.

Using proximity to ensure adequate speech input levels should not be limited to early infancy. All young cleft palate children should receive an audiological evaluation, and if slight hearing loss is shown to exist, arrangements should be made to have the child seated close to the teacher in school. In schools where activities or methods preclude formal seating arrangements, the teacher can usually find some way of being near the child during lessons. Too often the teacher is not made aware of the hearing problem or counselled on simple means of effectively teaching the child with a slight hearing loss. The responsibility for contacting the teacher may lie with the speech pathologist, the audiologist, or even the parent, but one member or another of the team must ensure that the contact is made.

While the effective use of proximity may be a sufficient means of ensuring adequate speech input for the child with slight hearing loss, children with impairment consistently averaging more than 25 dB (ISO) should be considered potential candidates for hearing aid use. Adults with vast experience of language and well-established listening skills begin to experience difficulty with hearing for speech when impairment exceeds 30 dB. For the child who has to acquire and develop language and listening skills, the critical level for intelligibility is lower than that for the adult. This is shown clearly by speech audiograms of children and adults: The shape of the articulation curve is much less steep for the former than for the latter.

Selection of an appropriate hearing aid for the child with mild to moderate conductive hearing loss poses no problem. Modern head-level hearing aids with electret microphones have a frequency range extending over several octaves, from below 200 Hz to above 5000 Hz, and sufficient gain to compensate for any conductive impairment. In most cases, the gain of the instrument selected should be about the same as the child's average hearing loss over the frequencies 500 to 2000 Hz. The maximum output should be well below the child's discomfort level, usually less than 115 dB. Where the child's comfortable listening level (MCL) is 100 dB or less, the earmold should be vented. For children with mild impairment (25 to 40 dB hearing levels) one hearing aid fitted to the poorer ear is usually adequate. For some with more severely impaired audition, two hearing aids rather than one might be required. Head-level hearing aids are preferable to body-worn instruments on several counts[52] and should, therefore, be given preference for those children who can be trained to wear them and treat them with a modicum of care. Earmolds should without exception be soft and flexible, since hard acrylic molds more readily cause damage when the child falls or receives a blow to the external ear.

Hearing and Listening

To hear is one thing: to listen, another. How well a person can listen and how well he does listen may be two different things. Children with hearing impairment, including those with cleft palate, tend to be much poorer listeners than their hearing deficit suggests they should be. Weaver[53] describes three aspects of listening: capacity, willingness, and habits, all of which may be affected by hearing loss. *Capacity* to listen concerns the ability to follow what is being said. Intelligence, knowledge of the subject, and previous experience in listening all contribute to this capacity. *Willingness* to listen may be selective or general. The child might want to listen in one situation, but not in another, or to one person, but not to another. On the other hand, he might be so concerned with talking (as some people are) that he rarely listens. *Habits* of listening exert a strong influence on ability to learn. A child quickly learns to "tune out" messages that are irrelevant to him, such as promises or threats which never materialize made by parents or speech which is constantly too difficult to hear.

Prevention and Remediation Programs

To prevent problems in language development from occurring is easier than to give remedial help when such problems have become established. The obvious time to initiate preventative measures is during the first few years of life, and the equally obvious people to carry out these measures are the parents.

Powers[54] recommends that early in the child's life the parents should be counselled concerning long-term plans and treatment in all potential problem areas. Since hearing loss is found in a large proportion of cases secondary to celft palate and, since it is possibly a major cause of language learning problems, parents should be informed that there is a strong possibility that it will affect their child. Further, parents should receive supportive counselling, starting as soon as hearing loss is diagnosed and continuing until successful management of the hearing problem is achieved.

The aims of the counselling program, which should be carried out by the audiologist and speech therapist in consultation with each other, would be to help the parents to (1) accept the facts and implications of hearing impairment secondary to the cleft palate problem; (2) acquire ability in speaking to their child at an appropriate distance and with an adequate voice level; (3) select a suitable hearing aid if the hearing loss reaches a chronic stage and is sufficiently severe, help them to learn to care for it, and help the child accept it; (4) encourage the child to develop the capacity, willingness, and habits fundamental to listening by offering pleasant and meaningful auditory experience; (5) persist in stimulating the child's efforts to communicate through speech; and (6) develop in themselves skills of observation so that they can report with accuracy the child's responses to sounds and attempts at speech.

The parents are really the key to successful early speech and language development, for they are present with the child during most of his early experience and a much greater part of his life at all times than the audiologist or speech therapist. It is they, not the therapist on a once-a-week basis, who can create and exploit natural and informal situations in everyday life making language more readily meaningful to a young child. It is they who have the opportunity to provide ideal opportunities for the child to develop not only good communication skills, but all-round integration of the child as an essential member of his family and society. It is they who must achieve consistently firm, but affectionate, handling of the child in a variety of situations promoting generally accepted standards of behavior and ability to compete and conform adequately in social situations. It is they who must also learn to meet the needs of the cleft palate child without jeopardising the well-being of the family as a whole. In all of this the audiologist, the speech therapist, and their co-workers must provide a guiding, supportive role. Therapists may be able to teach certain subskills of speech in the course of a series of once-a-week clinical visits, but the idea that they can alone teach a wide range of meaningful communication skills within such limited provision is ludicrous. Their role must essentially be that of mediating between the cleft palate child and his total environment, so that the conditions for his full development as a child are met. The type of program suggested is akin to the head start programs in which both children and their parents are helped to help themselves. Such programs should start not when the child has developed a language deficit, by the age of three or four, but before he has had a chance to do so. The intention is to prevent problems by helping the parents and others in the child's environment from the first signs of hearing loss, rather than to offer remedial help for an established problem.

There will always be a need for remedial therapy in certain cases, though many children currently receiving therapy are needing it only because of the benign neglect or ignorance of their earlier needs for preventative help. There will also be an increasing need, perhaps demand, for the evaluation of both parent guidance and remedial treatment programs. The literature on cleft palate includes few references to the evaluation of programs directly helping children with their communication skills and none to the evaluation of indirect therapy through parent guidance aimed at preventing language deficits. The areas of therapy with which we are concerned are expensive because they are time consuming, and increasing expenses lead to increasing the need for accountability. Without accountability based on evaluation and publications, the necessary funds for preventative and remedial therapy will not continue to be made available. It is true that the skills one should teach parents or children are hard to specify and to measure, but effectiveness in teaching these skills should be evaluated. If one claims they cannot be, then, as Mager[55] points out, one is in the awkward position of being unable to demonstrate that one is teaching anything at all. Charges have already been made that speech therapists tend to deal with the obvious speech problems of cleft palate children, to the exclusion of language problems more difficult to identify and remediate. Such charges should not generate feelings of hostility, but rather serve, as the writer hopes this chapter will, to stimulate audiologists and speech therapists to specify a wider range of feasible goals in their work, ways of achieving them, and methods of evaluating the extent to which both old and new objectives have been met.

REFERENCES

1. Skolnik, E.M.: Otologic evaluation in cleft palate patients. *Laryngoscope, 68*:1908-1949, 1958.
2. Masters, F.W., Bingham, H.G., and Robinson, D.W.: The prevention and treatment of hearing loss in the cleft palate child. *Plast. Reconstr Surg, 25*:503-509, 1960.
3. Spriestersbach, D.C., Lierle, D.M., Mill, K.L., and Prather, W.F.: Hearing loss in children with cleft palate. *Plast Reconstr Surg, 30*:336-347, 1962.
4. Walton, W.K.: Audiometrically "normal" conductive hearing losses among the cleft palate. *Cleft Palate J, 10*:99-103, 1973.
5. Shimo, G.: Middle ear problems associated with cleft palate. *Can J Otolaryngol, 1*:9-15, 1972.
6. Glover, D.M.: A long range evaluation of cleft palate repair. *Plast Reconstr Surg, 27*:19-30, 1961.
7. Hayes, C.S.: Audiological problems associated with cleft palate. *A.S.H.A. Rep, 1*:83-90, 1965.
8. Harrison, R.J. and Philips, B.J.: Observations of hearing levels of preschool cleft palate children. *J Speech Hear Disord, 36*:252-256, 1971.
9. Ling, D.: Rehabilitation of cases with deafness secondary to otitis media. In Glorig, A .and Gerwin, K.S. (Ed.): *Otitis Media.* Springfield, Thomas, 1972.
10. Ling, D., McCoy, R.H., and Levinson, E.D.: The incidence of middle ear disease and its educational implications among Baffin Island Eskimo children. *Can J Public Health, 60*:385-390, 1969.
11. Goetzinger, C.P.: Effects of small perceptual losses on language and on speech discrimination. *Volta Rev, 64*:408-412, 1967.
12. Goetzinger, C.P.: A study of hearing level and auditory discrimination of cleft palate adults. *Cleft Palate Bull, 10*:65-66, 1960.

13. Holm, V.A. and Kunze, L.H.: Effect of chronic otitis media on language and speech development. *Pediatrics, 43*:833-839, 1969.
14. Gaines, F.P.: Frequency and effect of hearing losses in cleft palate cases. *J Speech Hear Disord, 5*:141-149, 1940.
15. Eagles, E.L., Wishik, L.G., Doerfler, L.G., Melnick, W., and Levine, H.S.: Hearing sensitivity and related factors in children. *Laryngoscope* (Monogr. Suppl., June), 1963.
16. Baxter, J.D. and Ling, D.: Hearing loss among Baffin Zone Eskimos – A preliminary report. *Can J Otolaryngol, 1*:337-343, 1972.
17. Billig, A.L.: A psychological appraisal of cleft palate patients. *Proc Pa Acad Sci, 25*:29-31, 1951.
18. Illingworth, R.S. and Birch, L.B.: The intelligence of children with cleft palate. *Arch Dis Child, 31*:300-302, 1956.
19. Munson, S.E. and May, A.M.: Are cleft palate persons of subnormal intelligence? *J Educ Res, 48*:617-621, 1955.
20. Lewis, R.: A survey of the intelligence of cleft palate children in Ontario. *Cleft Palate Bull, 11*:83-85, 1961.
21. Means, B.J. and Irvin, J.: An analysis of certain measures of intelligence and hearing in a sample of the Wisconsin cleft palate population. *Cleft Palate Bull, 4*:4, 1954.
22. Ruess, A.L.: A comparative study of cleft palate children and their siblings. *J Clin Psychol, 21*:354-360, 1965.
23. Goodstein, L.D.: Intellectual impairment in children with cleft palates. *J Speech Hear Res, 4*:287-294, 1961.
24. Lamb, M.M., Wilson, F.B., and Leeper, H.A.: A comparison of selected cleft palate children and their siblings on the variables of intelligence, hearing loss, and visual-perceptual-motor abilities. *Cleft Palate J, 9*: 218-228, 1972.
25. Clifford, E.: Cleft palate and the person: Psychologic studies of its impact. *South Med J, 64*:1516-1520, 1971.
26. McWilliams, B.J.: Psychosocial development and modification. *A.S.H.A. Rep, 5*:165-187, 1970.
27. Birch, J.: Personality characteristics of individuals with cleft palate research needs. *Cleft Palate Bull, 2*:5-6, 1952.
28. Watson, C.G.: Personality adjustment in boys with cleft lips and palates. *Cleft Palate J, 1*:130-138, 1964.
29. Wirls, C.J. and Plotkin, R.R.: A comparison of children with cleft palate and their siblings on projective test personality factors. *Cleft Palate J, 8*:399-408, 1971.
30. Demb, N. and Ruess, A.L.: High school drop-out rate for cleft palate patients. *Cleft Palate J, 4*:327-333, 1967.
31. Smith, R.M. and McWilliams, B.J.: Creative thinking abilities of cleft palate children. *Cleft Palate J, 3*:275-283, 1966.
32. Bardach, J., Januszewska, W., and Jurzyk, R.: The social adaptation of

patients with cleft lip and palate. *Zdrow Publ, 81*:861-870, 1970.
33. McWilliams, B.J.: Speech and language problems in children with cleft palate. *J Am Med Wom Assoc, 21*:1005-1015, 1966.
34. Pannbacker, M.: Language skills of cleft palate children: A review. *Br J Disord Commun, 6*:37-44, 1971.
35. Bzoch, K.R.: A study of the speech of a group of pre-school cleft palate children. *Cleft Palate Bull, 9*:2-3, 1959.
36. Spriestersbach, D.C., Darley, F.L., and Morris, H.L.: Language skills in children with cleft palates. *J Speech Hear Res, 1*:279-285, 1958.
37. Morris, H.L.: Communication skills of children with cleft lips and palates. *J Speech Hear Res, 5*:79-90, 1962.
38. Nation, J.E.: Vocabulary comprehension and usage of pre-school cleft palate and normal children. *Cleft Palate J, 7*:639-644, 1970.
39. Smith, R.M. and McWilliams, B.J.: Psycholinguistic abilities of children with clefts. *Cleft Palate J, 5*:238-249, 1968.
40. Philips, B.J. and Harrison, R.J.: Language skills of preschool cleft palate children. *Cleft Palate J, 6,* 108-119, 1969.
41. Ebert, P.R.: *A Comparison of the Written Language Ability of Cleft Palate and Normal Children.* Unpublished dissertation, University of Pittsburgh (1968).
42. Templin, M.C.: *Certain Language Skills in Children.* Institute of Child Welfare Monograph Series, #26. Minneapolis, Minn Pr (1957).
43. Van Demark, D.R. and Van Demark, A.A.: Speech and socio-vocational aspects of individuals with cleft palate. *Cleft Palate J, 7*:284-299, 1970.
44. Westlake, H. and Rutherford, D.: *Cleft Palate.* Englewood Cliffs, Prentice-Hall, 1966.
45. Liberman, A.M., Cooper, F.S., Shankweiler, D.P., and Studdart-Kennedy, M.: Perception of the speech code. *Psychol Rev, 74*:431-461, 1967.
46. Menyuk, P.: Comparison of grammar of children with functionally deviant and normal speech. *J Speech Hear Res, 7*:109-121, 1964.
47. Lee, L. and Canter, S.M.: Developmental sentence scoring: A clinical procedure for estimating syntactic development in children's spontaneous speech. *J Speech Hear Res, 36*:315-340, 1971.
48. Galkowski, Y., Gassowski, P. and Grossman, J.: Influence of hearing disorders on development of speech in children with cleft lip palate. *Folia Phoniatr, 22*:72-78, 1970.
49. Nation, J.E.: Determinants of vocabulary development of preschool cleft palate children. *Cleft Palate J, 7*:645-651, 1970.
50. Goodstein, L.: MMPI differences between parents of children with cleft palates and parents of physically normal children. *J Speech Hear Res, 3*:31-38, 1960.
51. Smith, R.M. and McWilliams, B.J.: Psycholinguistic considerations in the management of children with cleft palate. *J Speech Hear Disord, 33*:27-33, 1968.

52. Ling, D.: Conventional hearing aids: An overview. *Volta Rev, 73*:343-352; 375-383, 1971.
53. Weaver, C.H.: *Human Listening: Processes and Behavior.* New York, Bobbs-Merrill Co., 1972.
54. Powers, G.R.: *Cleft Palate.* New York, Bobbs-Merrill Co., 1973.
55. Mager, R.F.: *Preparing Instructional Objectives.* Belmont, Fearon, 1962.

—9—

TYMPANIC MEMBRANE: NORMAL AND ABNORMAL

Richard A. Buckingham, M.D.

INTRODUCTION

Cleft palate patients, especially infants and children, should have careful, repeated, periodic, microscopic, otoscopic examinations to detect and prevent chronic ear disease and deafness. The otoscopic photographs in this chapter illustrate the necessity of otoscopic surveillance.

The nature of the congenital defect resulting in cleft palate also affects the opening and closing mechanism of the eustachian tube. The alteration of the opening and closing of the eustachian tube causes malfunction of the eustachian tube and poor middle ear aeration, which in turn leads to serous otitis media, atelectasis, chronic adhesive otitis media, and eventually, to cholesteatoma formation.

Not all cleft palate patients suffer from eustachian malfunction, but because many of them do, they must all be carefully followed.

Normal Tympanic Membrane

Plate 3-1 is a photograph of a normal right tympanic membrane. The anatomical structures are indicated in the diagram accompanying the photograph (Figure 9-1).

The malleus handle lies toward the center of the photograph. The short process of the malleus lies superiorly, and the umbo

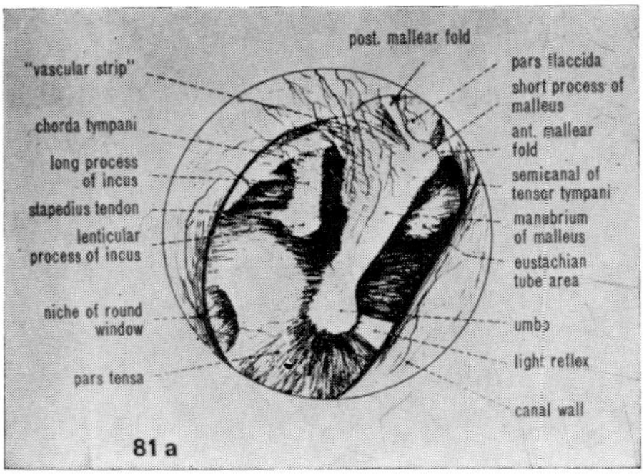

Figure 9-1. Diagram of tympanic membrane in Color illustration 1, Plate 3.

forms the inferior extremity of the malleus handle.

In this ear the pars tensa is translucent, and some of the structures within the middle ear can be visualized through the membrane.

The long process of the incus is discernible posterosuperiorly. The stapedius tendon stretches posteriorly from the stapes neck at the inferior extremity of the long process of the incus.

The promontory of the cochlea lies posteriorly at the level of the umbo. The round window niche appears as the dark shadow lying at the posterior edge of the photograph, just below the level of the umbo.

In cases of cleft palate, the otologist must first determine if the ear is normal or abnormal. He looks for the normal landmarks of the tympanic membrane as demonstrated in Plate 3-1 and Figure 9-1. He studies the membrane for retracted or atelectatic areas. He tries to see through the membrane to determine if the middle ear is aerated normally or if there is fluid or mucus present within. When the tympanic membrane is normal and the middle ear is well aerated in a cleft palate patient, the clinician is safe in assuming that the patient has normal hearing even if he is too young for an accurate audiogram. A normally aerated middle ear indicates that eustachian tube function is normal. The visualization of normal tympanic membrane and a well-aerated middle ear is perhaps the best test of eustachian tube function available today.

To diagnose a normal tympanic membrane, the ear should be examined through the Zeiss® operating microscope. Children require very delicate and careful handling during the examination of the ear. Wax and debris must be carefully and gently removed from the external canal before the tympanic membrane can be seen. In infants and small children, small (even minute) specula must be used because of the small size of the external auditory canal. The tympanic membrane of the newborn is the same size as that of the adult, but the tympanic membrane of the infant lies in an almost horizontal position and the external auditory canal is shorter and narrower than in the adult. When there is an associated stenosis of the external auditory canal, examination of the tympanic membrane may be impossible. In infants and small children the tympanic membrane becomes hyperemic and reddened when the child cries or screams. Therefore, if at all possible, the tympanic membrane should be visualized with the child at rest.

The middle ear and tympanic membrane of a cleft palate patient may appear normal at first examination. However, repeated examinations should be made at intervals of two to four times yearly during infancy and childhood to study the ear under different conditions. It is important to know the status of the ear during and following upper respiratory infections. If serious

---

Plate 3-1. Normal right tympanic membrane.

Plate 3-2. Acute otitis media, right.

Plate 3-3. Serous otitis media, right.

Plate 3-4. Serous otitis media, left.

Plate 3-5. Glue-type otitis serous media, right.

Plate 3-6. Same ear as Plate 3-5, glue partially removed.

Plate 3-8. Same ear as Plates 3-5, 3-6, and 3-7 several months later, tube in place.

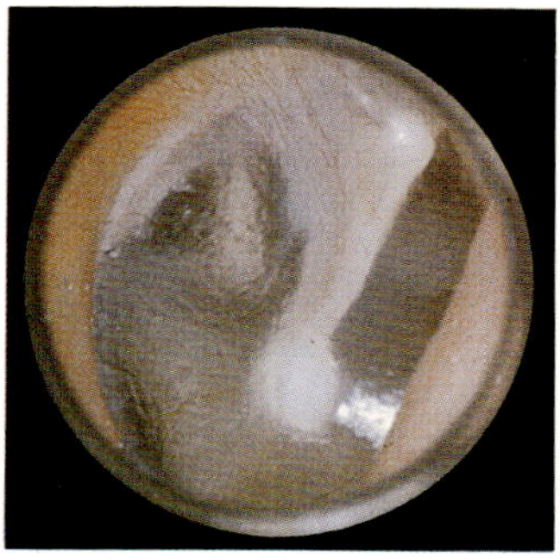
Plate 3-1.

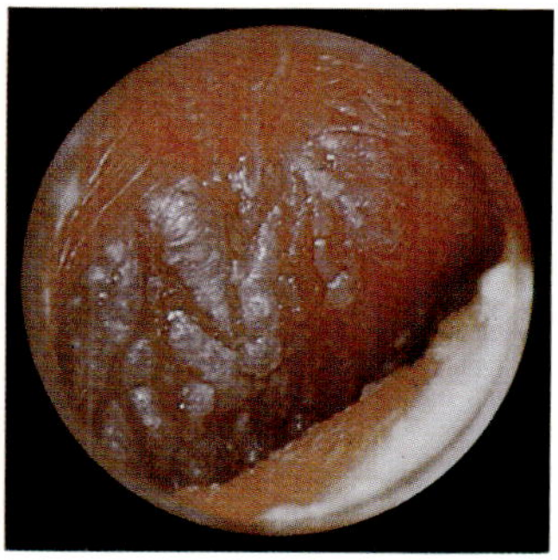
Plate 3-2.

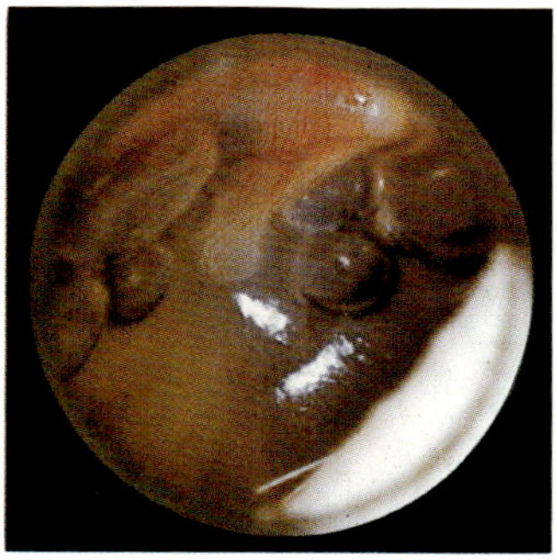
Plate 3-3.

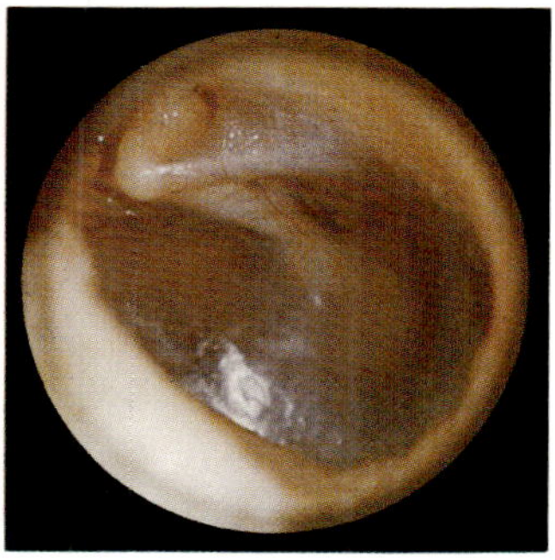
Plate 3-4.

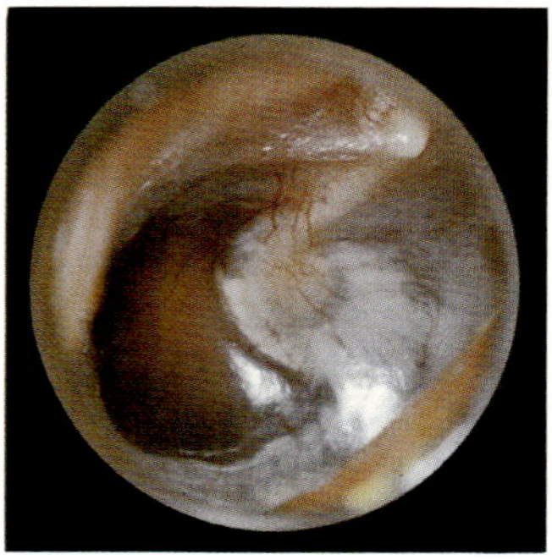
Plate 3-5.

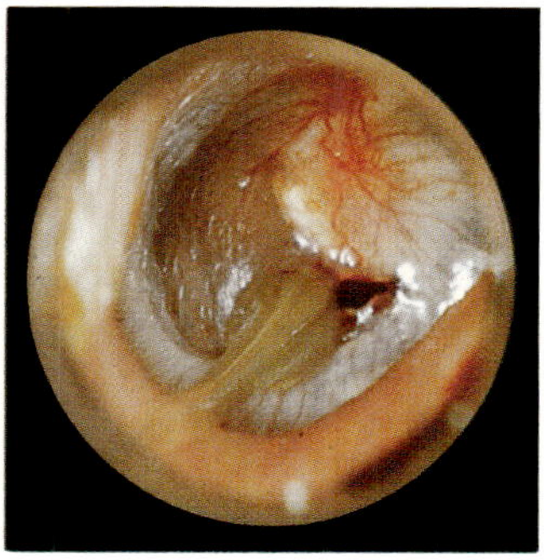
Plate 3-6.

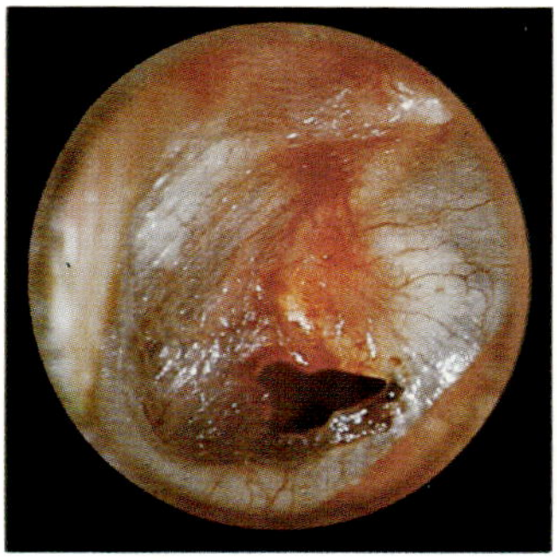
Plate 3-7.

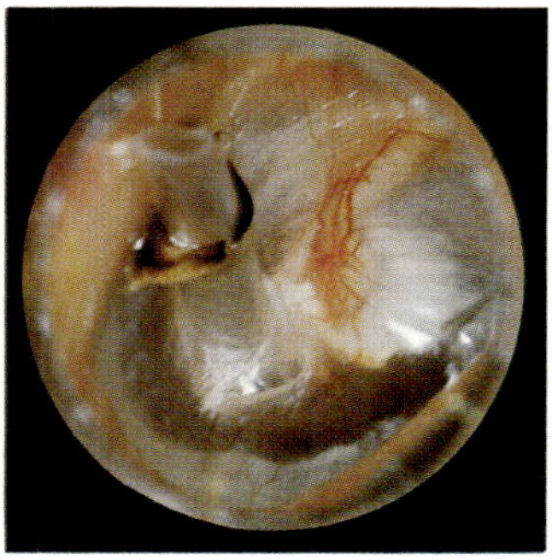
Plate 3-8.

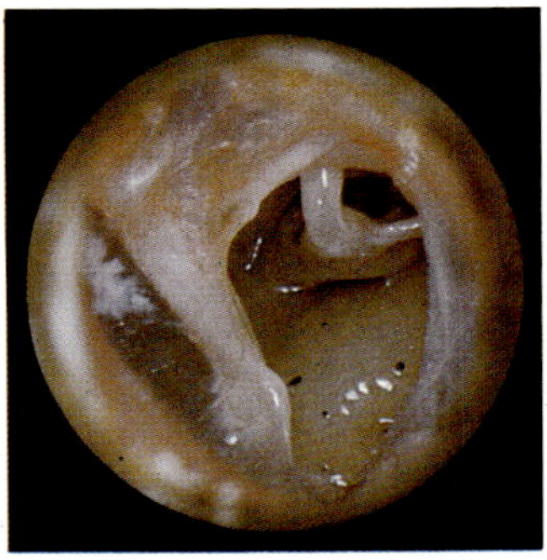

Plate 4-1.

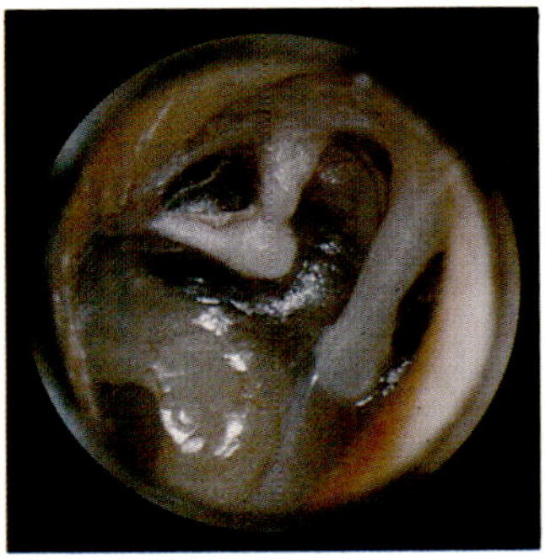

Plate 4-2.

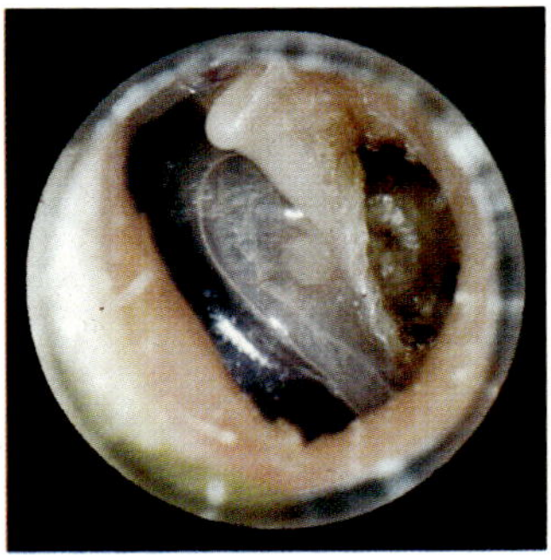

Plate 4-3.

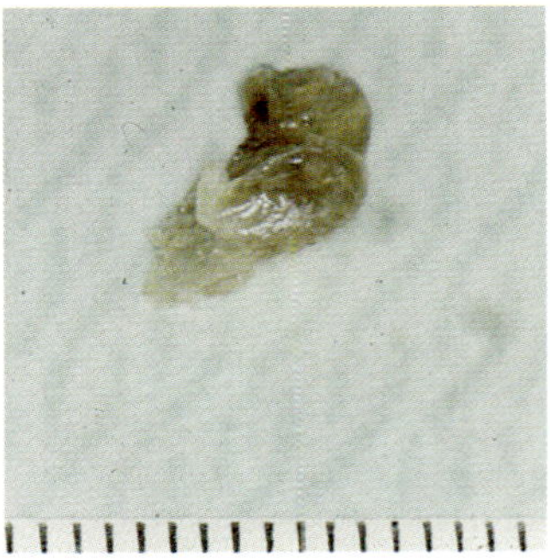

Plate 4-4.

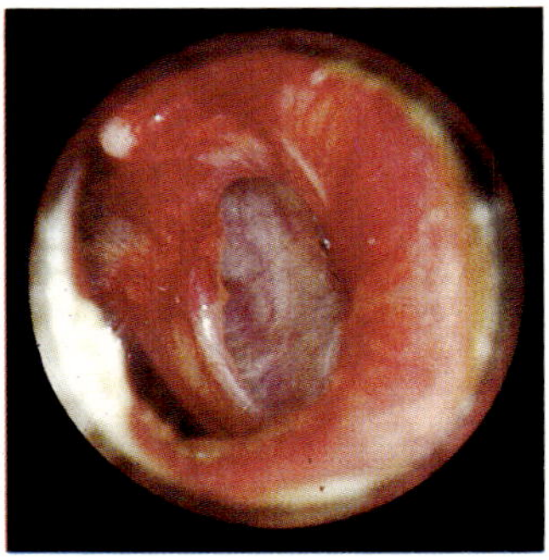

Plate 4-5.

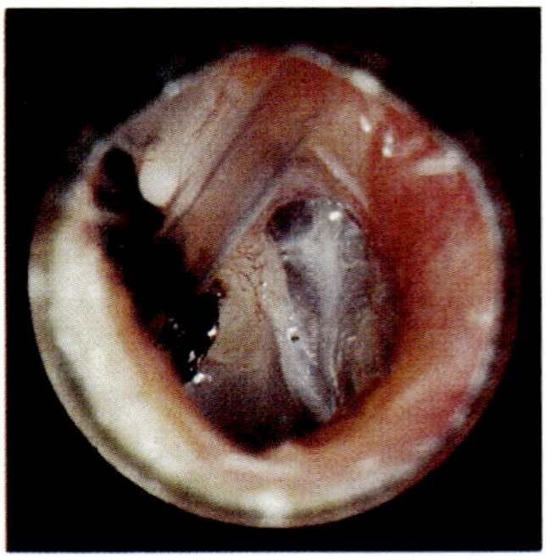

Plate 4-6.

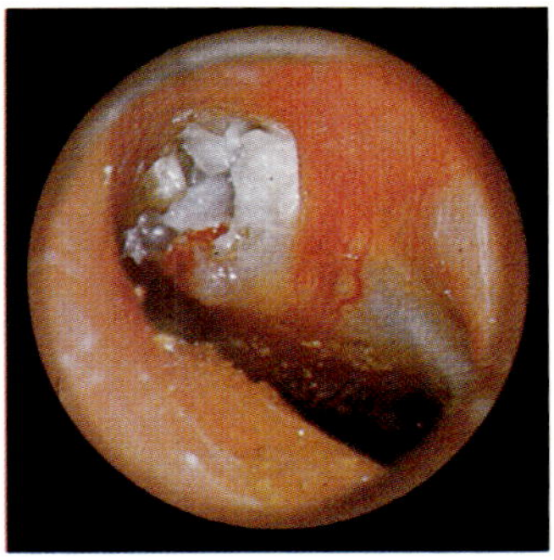

Plate 4-7.

trouble is to develop in the ears of the cleft palate patient, it will most likely occur as a result of an upper respiratory infection extending into the middle ears.

It is possible for serious pathology to develop in the ear of a child with a cleft palate without external signs, pain, discharge, or even without hearing loss.

In the author's rather limited experience, approximately 50 percent of all children with cleft palate have normal tympanic membranes on the first and subsequent examinations. The other 50 percent show signs of some kind of tympanic membrane pathology at one time or another over a prolonged period of observation.

In those few cases with normal tympanic membranes and middle ears but with audiometric findings of conductive deafness, the cause will most likely be a congenital abnormality of the ossicular chain or of the oval window.

Acute Otitis Media

Plate 3-2 shows the typical otoscopic appearance of an ear with acute otitis media.

The normal landmarks of the tympanic membrane are absent, and even the malleus short process is obliterated.

The entire tympanic membrane is reddened, and the mem-

Plate 4-1. Central perforation of tympanic membrane, left.

Plate 4-2. Chronic adhesive otitis media, right.

Plate 4-3. Cholesteatoma, posterior superior marginal type, left.

Plate 4-4. Cholesteatoma nidus from Plate 4-3.

Plate 4-5. Same ear as Plate 4-3, following nidus removal.

Plate 4-6. Same ear as Plates 4-3 and 4-5 several months later, tube in place.

Plate 4-7. Cholesteatoma, attic type, left.

The otoscopic photographs are from W. Becker, R.A. Buckingham, P.H. Holinger, G.W. Korting, and F.L. Lederer: Atlas of Otothinolaryngology and Bronchoesophagology, 1970. Courtesy of W.B. Saunders Company, Philadelphia.

brane bulges laterally due to the presence of inflammatory exudate under increased pressure within the middle ear.

In cases of repeated, recurrent acute otitis, this lateral herniation and inflammation probably results in dissolution of the middle, fibrous layer of the tympanic membrane. With resolution of the acute otitis the site of the dissolution of the fibrous layer appears as an atrophic, thin, easily retracted area in the pars tensa, as seen in Plates 3-5 through 3-8.

Cleft palate patients do not seem to be more susceptible to acute otitis media than those children with normal palates.

The treatment of acute otitis media in the cleft palate patient should be the same as in the normal child.

Tonsillectomy and adenoidectomy are usually interdicted in cleft palate patients, and therefore, they are spared this rather questionable form of therapy for recurrent acute otitis media.

Serous Otitis Media

Plates 3-3 and 3-4 are otoscopic photographs of ears with serous otitis media.

The air bubbles seen through the tympanic membrane in Plate 3-3 indicate that this middle ear is partially aerated. The air bubbles can be recognized by their rounded appearance, their lighter color, and by the air-fluid interface which demarcates the fluid from the air-filled areas in the middle ear.

The presence of the air bubbles in the middle ear increases the contrast between the fluid and air-filled portions of the middle ear, and simplifies the diagnosis of serous otitis.

In Plate 3-4 the entire middle ear is filled with dark, yellow-tinged serous fluid, and there is no air-filled space remaining. This otoscopic appearance is far more common in serous otitis than that seen in Plate 3-3. When the middle ear is completely filled with serous fluid, the otoscopic diagnosis is difficult and may be missed. When there is no air-fluid interface, the examiner must look through the translucent tympanic membrane to see the fluid within the middle ear. The otoscopic microscope is the best instrument to visualize fluid in the middle ear.

There are ancillary findings of serous otitis in the tympanic membrane in Plate 3-4 that help to confirm the diagnosis. These ancillary findings are caused by negative or underpressure in the middle ear and the yellow color of the fluid.

Negative pressure causes an indrawing of the tympanic membrane. As the membrane is drawn medially, the attached malleus handle, too, is drawn medially. Because the axis of rotation of the malleus is eccentric, the handle moves upward and backward. The result of this upward and backward movement is an apparent optical shortening of the malleus handle. The indrawing of the malleus handle causes the short process of the malleus to rotate externally. Hence, in serous otitis, the short process of the malleus handle appears more prominent than normal.

The inward retraction of the tympanic membrane and the outward projection of the short process of the malleus cause the posterior mallear fold to become more prominent than normal. In Plate 3-4, the posterior mallear fold is very prominent.

The prominence of the posterior mallear fold in Plate 3-4 is best seen when a comparison is made of this photograph with the normal tympanic membrane in Plate 3-1.

The pars flaccida is retracted in serous otitis media because this area of the tympanic membrane lacks a middle, fibrous layer. The retraction of the pars flaccida is apparent in Plate 3-4.

Because of the yellow color of the fluid within the middle ear, the bone of the malleus handle in serous otitis media appears by contrast to have a chalky whiteness, which is seen in Plate 3-4.

Serous otitis is the most common ear disorder associated with cleft palates. One author[2] found that 97 percent of cleft palate children have serous otitis. When it occurs in noncleft palate patients, serous otitis media is most probably caused by eustachian tube malfunction. Since a cleft palate affects the opening and closing mechanism of the eustachian tube, it is easy to understand why cleft palate patients are so often affected by serous otitis media.

The origin of the serous fluid itself is from mucous– and serous– secreting glands that lie on the medial wall of the middle ear.[5] Since serous otitis media occurs during, preceding, or following an acute upper respiratory infection, the congenital defect of the opening and closing musculature of the eustachian tube, plus the inflammation of the upper respiratory infection are assumed to combine somehow in the pathogenesis of serous otitis.

In some cleft palate patients with serous otitis, allergy plays a role, too, in the etiology of serous otitis media, but allergy is another form of inflammation. Many cleft palate patients have serous otitis media without having any allergies.

The part hypertrophic adenoids play in the causation of serous otitis media in cleft and in noncleft palate patients has not been definitely determined.

Until recently adenoidectomy in cleft palate patients was absolutely forbidden, so that it has not been possible to observe if the serous otitis media would clear up following adenoidectomy. With the development of the pharyngeal flap, adenoidectomy may be indicated in some cleft palate patients before the flap procedure to remove a large mass of lymphoid tissue in the nasopharynx. It is the author's personal opinion that adenoidectomy is not a specific curative treatment for serous otitis.

Serous otitis media may resolve spontaneously in cleft and noncleft palate patients. For persistent and nonresolved serous otitis, the treatment is middle ear aeration with a middle ear vent, as described by Armstrong[1].

Incising the tympanic membrane, aspirating the fluid, and aerating the middle ear with a polyethylene tube will restore the ear to the normal aerated state in most cases of serous otitis media.

Since the effect of the middle ear aeration with the tube is to equalize middle ear and external atmosphere pressures, it is difficult to deny that the chief factor in the pathogenesis of serous otitis is negative middle ear pressure.

Negative middle ear pressure in serous otitis media can be measured directly with a minimanometer[3] or directly by impedance audiometry.[4]

It is not necessary to intubate every case of serous otitis media in patients with cleft palate. It will be seen, however, in Plates 4-3 through 4-6 that negative middle ear pressure in certain ears, with or without serous fluid, may lead to cholesteatoma formation.

Therefore, in these cases of cleft palate with serous otitis and signs of marked negative middle ear pressure and deep localized or generalized tympanic membrane retraction, prompt middle ear intubation is indicated.

Serous Otitis Media, Glue Ear Type

Plates 3-5 through 3-8 demonstrate the otoscopic findings and treatment in an ear with the glue type of serous otitis media.

The typical otoscopic findings of serous otitis media are present in Plate 3-5. The posterior half of the tympanic membrane is thin, atrophic, and void of a middle fibrous area. Because the atrophic area is so thin, it is easy to appreciate the presence of dark, yellow-colored fluid within the middle ear. This thin atrophic area is retracted medially due to the negative middle ear pressure often associated with serous otitis media. The anterior half and a thin posterior inferior segment of the pars tensa of the tympanic membrane have a white gray appearance because the middle layer is still present in this portion of the tympanic membrane.

The short process of the malleus projects laterally, the posterior mallear fold is prominent, and the malleus handle appears shorter than normal.

Plate 3-6 is a photograph of the same ear as Plate 3-5 following a myringotomy and partial aspiration of the gluey mucus found within the middle ear. The myringotomy incision lies inferiorly, and the lumen is filled with a strand of stringy mucus which stretches laterally and lies on the floor of the external auditory canal.

Plate 3-7 is the appearance of the same ear as Plate 3-5 and 3-6 after all of the gluey mucus has been aspirated. The myringotomy opening is about 1 $\times$ 2 mm in size, and the middle ear seen through this opening is free of fluid.

The posterior atrophic portion of the tympanic membrane which was retracted and atelectatic in Plate 3-5 has now expanded laterally to occupy the normal position of the membrane. The prominent posterior mallear fold has disappeared as the inward pull on the membrane has been relieved.

Plate 3-8 is the appearance of the same ear as in Plates 3-5, 3-6, and 3-7 several months later. The polyethylene middle ear air vent present in the posterior-inferior portion of the tympanic membrane has been in place since the myringotomy.

The middle ear is now aerated and the tympanic membrane expanded. Looking through the atrophic portion of the tympanic membrane with the Zeiss operating microscope, the observer can see that there is no fluid within the middle ear.

The origin of the glue found in this form of serous otitis media is from mucous glands that Lim[5] demonstrated, which line the medial wall of the middle ear.

It is not known why gluey mucus occurs in some ears with serous otitis media instead of the more common serous fluid.

Otoscopically, it is difficult or impossible to differentiate gluey from serous fluid within the middle ear before myringotomy. Through the operating microscope, the gluey mucus has a paler, less yellow appearance than serous fluid.

A myringotomy and polyethylene tube insertion is usually necssary to treat the glue-type serous otitis media because the glue type does not resolve spontaneously as often as the serous fluid type.

Both the glue and ordinary type of serous otitis media result in a conductive type hearing loss of variable degree.

Chronic Otitis Media with Central Perforation of Tympanic Membrane

Plate 4-1 shows a large, dry noninflamed central perforation of the posterior half of the left tympanic membrane.

The long process of the incus lies in the posterosuperior portion of the middle ear. The anterior and posterior crura of the stapes are visible anterior and posterior to the lenticular process of the incus. The stapedius tendon stretches posteriorly from the neck of the stapes.

The promontory of the medial wall of the middle ear lies inferior to the stapes.

The anterior margin of the perforation lies on the posterior border to the malleus handle. There is a narrow rim of intact pars tensa peripheral to the entire circumference of the perforation.

This narrow rim of intact pars tensa surrounding the edge of the perforation differentiates this central perforation from a marginal perforation. Marginal perforations extend to the bony rim of the tympanic annulus and do not have any pars tensa at the site of contact of the perforation rim with the bony annular rim. Marginal perforations are often associated with cholesteatomas of the middle ear and mastoid.

While the cause of central perforations such as this is presumed to be a single attack of acute otitis media, the spontaneous perforation which occurs in acute otitis media, in an otherwise normal tympanic membrane, is usually a small pinpoint area. Large perforations of the size seen in Plate 4-1 probably occur following an attack of recurrent otitis media in atrophic areas of the tympanic membrane caused by repeated, antecedent bouts of acute otitis media. In central perforations without scarring or inflammation and with an intact ossicular chain, the hearing may often be normal.

In a cleft palate patient, if a central perforation of the type shown in Plate 4-1 is closed by myringoplasty, inadequate eustachian tube function and negative middle ear pressure can lead to atelectasis of the tympanic membrane graft and to beginning cholesteatoma formation. Following a successful myringoplasty in a cleft palate patient, the surgeon may find himself in the paradoxical situation of having to make a new perforation for a polyethylene tube in the recently repaired tympanic membrane to relieve atelectasis.

Chronic Adhesive Otitis Media

Plate 4-2 and the accompanying diagram, Figure 9-2, show the otoscopic findings in a right ear with chronic adhesive otitis media. The posterior half of the tympanic membrane is thin and atrophic. Because of negative middle ear pressure, this thin, atrophic portion of the tympanic membrane has collapsed medially to form an atelectatic middle ear. Posterosuperiorly, the atrophic membrane lies in contact with and partially envelopes the long process of the incus, stapes head and stapedius tendon. Inferiorly, the atelectatic membrane lies in contact with the promontory.

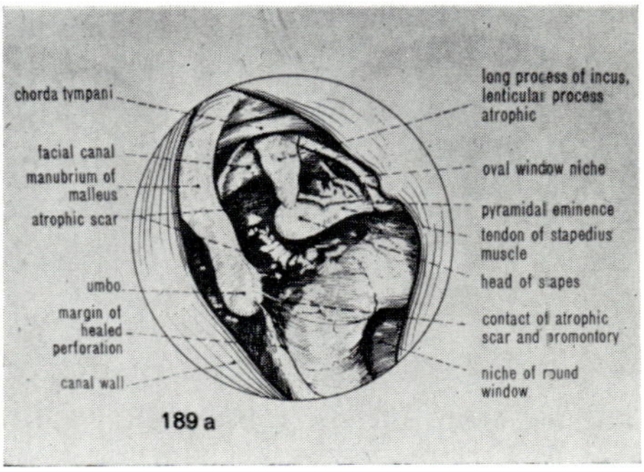

Figure 9-2. Diagram of chronic adhesive otitis media in Color Illustration 10, Plate 4.

In this particular ear, the ossicular chain was fixed by fibrosis in the epitympanum. Probably in this type of atrophic, atelectatic tympanic membrane, an attack of acute otitis media would result in the slough of the atrophic membrane and in a perforation of the type seen in Plate 4-1.

Cholesteatoma, Posterosuperior Marginal Perforation Type, Early, Reversible

Plates 4-3 through 4-6 show the otoscope findings in a small cholesteatoma of the posterosuperior marginal type. Fortunately for the patient, this cholesteatoma was small and had not eroded the ossicular chain. Local therapy with middle ear polyethylene tube aeration and removal of the epithelial debris resulted in the reversal of the pathological process and in the disappearance of the cholesteatoma. These photographs demonstrate the role of the eustachian tube malfunction, middle ear atelectasis, and epithelial debris accumulation in the pathogenesis cholesteatoma.

Plate 4-3 shows the appearance of the patient when first seen. There is a posterosuperior marginal-type perforation filled with dried, necrotic, epithelial debris. The tympanic membrane shows the typical appearance of a cholesteatoma of the pars tensa. Anterior to the malleus handle and umbo, within the middle ear, there is a forward extension of the cholesteatoma cyst lying in contact with the medial wall of the tympanic membrane.

This ear was treated first with daily installations of Terra-

Cortril Ear Suspension® for two to three weeks. This medication has an oil base which softened the core or nidus of epithelial debris lying within the lumen of the cholesteatoma.

Plate 4-4 shows the nidus of epithelial debris removed through the lumen of the posterosuperior marginal perforation.

Plate 4-5 shows the appearance of the tympanic membrane seen in Plate 4-3 immediately following removal of the epithelial nidus. There appears to be a posterior marginal perforation whose anterior margin extends inferiorly from the malleus handle toward the posterior bony margin of the tympanic annulus.

All procedures in this ear were done with the aid of the Zeiss operating microscope. With the microscope, it was clear that the medial wall of this perforation was actually an atelectatic, stretched inpocketed, atrophic tympanic membrane continuous with the tympanic membrane through the entire circumference of the posterior marginal perforation.

This perforation was not a true perforation, but a rather deep and extensive blind sinus whose mouth was the apparent perforation.

In Plate 4-6 the end result of middle ear ventilation with a polyethylene tube is seen. This is the same ear as Plates 4-3 and 4-5. The negative pressure in the middle ear was equalized with the middle ear vent, and the atelectatic, stretched tympanic membrane gradually shrank and tightened up over a period of several months.

In Plate 4-6 this atrophic posterior portion of the tympanic membrane has finally expanded laterally to the level of the normal tympanic membrane. Since the ossicular chain was not eroded, the hearing in this patient, which was normal when he was first seen, remained so throughout the course of treatment.

The patient shown here did not have a cleft palate, but poor eustachian tube function is undoubtedly the cause of many cholesteatomas of this type in cleft palate patients.

Cholesteatoma, Attic, Pars Flaccida Type, Far Advanced

Plate 4-7 shows a perforation in the pars flaccida or attic area of the left ear. The lumen of the perforation is filled with epithelial debris. The short process of the malleus is visible at the inferior margin of the perforation. The intact pars tensa of the tympanic membrane extends inferiorly. This patient has an extensive cholesteatoma of the middle ear and mastoid process.

This ear demonstrates the end result of unrelieved eustachian tube malfunction and inflammation. This ear cannot be treated conservatively, and extensive surgery is necessary to treat the cholesteatoma.

The problem with pars flaccida cholesteatoma is that retraction of the pars flaccida extends into the epitympanum lateral to the ossicular chain behind the bony cover of the lateral epitympanic wall. In this hidden region, an incipient cholesteatoma cannot be discovered as it can in aetelectatic areas of the pars tensa. Attic cholesteatomas are usually well developed before the otologist can diagnose them.

In cleft palate patients, as in all other patients with serous otitis media, atelectasis, or other signs of eustachian tube malfunction, the tympanic membrane, both pars flaccida or pars tensa, should be studied carefully with the Zeiss operating microscope. When localized atelectatic areas are noted in the pars tensa, or when the pars flaccida becomes retracted, the middle ear should be aerated with a polyethylene tube to relieve negative middle ear pressure and to allow the atelectatic portion of the tympanic membrane to expand.

Summary

In this chapter the author has shown otoscopic photographs of several different pathological conditions of the ear occurring commonly in patients with cleft palate.

While the photographs shown here are not taken from cleft palate patients, the pathology in the noncleft palate and the cleft palate patient is the same. The underlying etiology in most chronic ear disorders is eustachian tube malfunction, and unfortunately, this malfunction affects both cleft palate and noncleft palate patients.

Since cleft palate patients are known to have a high incidence of eustachian tube malfunction, it is essential for the clinician to follow these patients carefully from birth to maturity, and even later. Periodic, microscopic otoscopic examination is the only way that early changes in the tympanic membrane can be recognized. When early atelectasis or cholesteatoma formation is noted, middle ear aeration and proper local therapy can prevent irreversible, disabling, pathologic alterations of the middle ear.

Audiometric checks should be made periodically, but it is important to realize that in an ear, such as Plates 4-3, 4-4, 4-5, and 4-6 pathologic changes can be fairly well advanced with minimal or no changes in the audiometric thresholds.

In Plate 4-3, the nidus of the cholesteatoma did not interfere with sound conduction. Had this patient been followed by audiometric tests only, irreversible changes would surely have occurred before anything untoward would have been noted autometrically.

The cleft palate patient has many extra handicaps in addition to the cleft palate. One of these additional handicaps is a propensity for ear disease due to poor eustachian tube function. Careful periodic microscopic otoscopy is mandatory, or permanent deafness will become an added handicap.

REFERENCES

1. Armstrong, B.W.: A new treatment for chronic secretory otitis media. *Arch Otolaryngol, 59:*653-654, 1954.
2. Bluestone, C.D.: Eustachian tube obstruction in the infant with cleft palate. *Ann Otol Rhinol Laryngol, 80:*Supplement no. 2, 1972.
3. Buckingham, R.A. and Ferrer, J.L.: Middle ear pressures in eustachian tube malfunction, manometric studies. *Laryngoscope, 80:*1585-1593, 1973.
4. Harford, E.R.: Tympanometry for eustachian tube evaluation. *Arch Orolaryngol, 97:*17-20, 1973.
5. Lim, D.J. and Shimada, T.: Secretory activity of normal middle ear epithelium. *Ann Otol Rhinol Laryngol, 80:*319-329, 1971.

Author Index

Subject Index

G

H

I

N